GENTLE DENTAL

FACING DENTAL FEAR

DEDICATION

To my clients, whose courage and faith ...

ACKNOWLEDGEMENTS

I would like to thank my partner, Stuart Gibson, MSc, for his considerable and sustaining insight, wisdom, experience and support, both personal and professional, throughout the genesis of this book.

NOTE

The stories contained within these pages are true. All client names and certain details have been changed to protect confidentiality.

ABOUT THE AUTHOUR

Dr Kathy Nathan is an award winning dentist, teacher, researcher, author and speaker with over three decades of experience in NHS and private general dental practice in Australia and the UK. She qualified as a dentist with additional science honours in 1984, and gained the diploma and membership of the Faculty of General Dental Practitioners, Royal College of Surgeons in 1996. She is the founder of Gentle Dental in Harrow and works in Centre of Dental Excellence caring for people with dental anxiety and phobias. She lives in north London with her partner, a psychotherapist, and their two daughters.

SHARE THE LOVE

Please tell me your inspiring stories of overcoming dental fear and phobias so that they might be included in future editions of Gentle Dental. To share your experiences and feedback, visit my website at www.gentledentalharrow.co.uk
and e-mail via links to info@centreofdentalexcellence.co.uk.

CONTENTS

WHY DID I WRITE THIS BOOK?
HOW THIS BOOKS WORKS.

PART ONE: IS THIS BOOK FOR YOU?

Chapter 1. Do you have a dental phobia?

Chapter 2. You are not alone.

Chapter 3. A better way forward.

Chapter 4. Why bother?

Chapter 5. Is dental phobia treatable?

PART TWO: YOUR PERSONAL **SMILE!** PLAN

Chapter 6. Select your smile supporters.

Choose your support team.
Choose your dentist.

Chapter 7. Make an appointment.

Making a decision to trust.
Taking a leap of faith.
Taking Action.
Celebration.

Chapter 8. Indulge in self-care.

GENERAL WELLBEING
MENTAL WELLBEING
DENTAL WELLBEING

Chapter 9. Lift off! Visit your dentist.

FIND YOUR FEARS, FIX YOUR PHOBIAS:
General fears.
Dental fears.
Chapter 10. Enjoy! Review, Repeat, Reward.

RESOURCES

INDEX
WHY DID I WRITE THIS BOOK?

Over the last thirty years I have developed a particular interest in caring for people, who, like myself, entertain a perfectly understandable and healthy disrespect for dentists and dentistry to a greater or lesser degree. Using specific carefully researched skills and techniques, I have been privileged to share the love and transform the smiles and lives of thousands of such terrified people with often self-proclaimed 'terrible teeth'.

My personal journey in facing dental fear began in early childhood. As a toddler, I was weaned on sweetened milk and sugary food. The fillings in my decayed baby teeth were provided impersonally and without anaesthetic. I did not like going to the dentist. My first clear memory of going to the dentist was in Adelaide, the Australian city where I grew up.

This dentist's clinic consisted of a single tiny room in an imposing office block on the most prestigious street in the city centre. I was about eleven years of age. An efficient dental nurse collected me from the waiting room and walked me down the corridor to the surgery. The dentist was slim, silver haired and business like.

'Sit yourself down,' he said, indicating the dental chair.

I did what I was told.

The nurse anchored a disposable bib on my chest with a metal chain at the back of my neck and small alligator clips. She picked up a paper chart and a pen.

'Upper right seven partly erupted,' the dentist began. The nurse scribbled away.

'Ot aah oo oing?' I asked, my mouth wide open.

My new dentist paused momentarily, taking his instruments out of my mouth.

'I'm checking your teeth. Isn't that why you're here?' he asked.

'What's an upper right seven?' I asked.

I continued to ask questions, feeling anxious and vulnerable in this unfamiliar situation.

'Let's get on, shall we?' my new dentist finally said.

'Will you stop if I raise my hand?' I asked, making one last effort to maintain control.

'No, I won't,' the dentist said. 'I'm only going to do what I'm going to do anyway and I can't keep stopping for questions.'

He raised his instruments expectantly and I opened my mouth again. He carried on counting and charting my teeth. Cleaning, oral hygiene instruction and a fluoride treatment followed. Later, he placed a couple of white fillings in my front teeth. It felt uncomfortable on my sensitive incisors. I survived, with a continued dislike of dental visits.

These days, I am much improved, probably because I am now a dentist myself. I am better at choosing skilled and empathic dental care givers and I have won excellent mileage from my teeth and gums, with much less trauma, as a result. I still occasionally get anxious, especially when seeing someone new. I consider a raised hand 'stop signal' my minimum requirement for comfort.

And, as I have come to realize, I am not alone. Many people experience similar or far worse dental and life challenges than mine. This book is offered in the hope that within its pages lie the means for all of us to secure good, safe, comfortable dental care and perhaps, just as importantly, to feel better about ourselves, our smiles, and sometimes, maybe, even our dentists.

HOW THIS BOOKS WORKS

GENTLE DENTAL is a toolkit for those of us blessed with dental fears and phobias. It is designed to get us to our dentists, give us a good enough time when we're there, and gift us with glorious grins at the end of it all.

It's also an inspiring source of information and motivation for those of us who relish true tales of ordinary folk overcoming isolation, tragedy and terror to reap togetherness, triumph and truly magnificent teeth - especially if we would like to number ourselves amongst them.

After you have read Part One you will know if **GENTLE DENTAL** is for you. You will also know that you are not alone, that you too can visit the dentist and enjoy better health and confidence, and that your beautiful smile is both a reward in itself and the gift that goes on giving to others.

Then, as you read Part Two, you will discover the five simple **SMILE!** steps that will help you triumph over your dental fears and phobias:

1. Select your support team and dentist.

Choose the right people to cheer you on in your smile care challenge.

2. Make an appointment.

Find the courage to visit that website, write that email, pick up that phone and do whatever it takes to reserve an appointment with your chosen dentist.

3. Indulge in self-care.

Screen yourself for general, mental and dental wellbeing, and begin a program of loving self-care as you prepare for your first dental visit.

4. Lift off!

Discover handy ways to manage all kinds of fears and phobias at your dental visit. Go for it!

5. Enjoy!

Review your visit, keep up the good work, reward yourself, and **SMILE!**

Are you sitting comfortably? Let us begin…

PART ONE

IS THIS BOOK FOR YOU?

Chapter 1. Do you have a dental phobia?

Are you an anxious, nervous, fearful and phobic dental patient?

The aim of this book is to help us feel better about ourselves, our smiles and maybe even our dentists. Many alarmingly explicit and complicated dental questionnaires exist to measure dental anxiety and are often used for research. But for our purposes, to affirm ourselves, our fears and our phobias, the following questionnaire is more than sufficient. Us dental dodgers and dislikers know who we are…

DENTAL PHOBIA QUESTIONNAIRE:

ASK YOURSELF…

- Do you 'hate the dentist'?

- Has your confidence, health, career or relationships suffered as a result of avoiding dental care?

- Do you only go to the dentist when you are in pain?

- Do you make dental appointments that you fail to keep?

- Do you have difficulty sleeping the night before a dental appointment?

- Have you ever walked out during a dental appointment or failed to complete a course of dental treatment?

If you answered, '**Yes**', to any one of the above questions, congratulations! * Chances are you have a good old-fashioned gold plated dental phobia. Maybe more than one. Even if you're not sure, even if you do go regularly, but perhaps experience mild trepidation and dislike of the dentist and all the strange and wonderful things they do, this book will help put your fears into perspective and give you the knowledge and confidence you need to enjoy your visits.

* Why congratulations? Because you now know more about yourself. Awareness is the first step in making positive changes in your life, if you choose to do so.

Chapter 2. You are not alone.

If you are dentally fearful or phobic, you are not alone. Around a third of us fear dental visits. Almost half of us with anxiety don't go regularly and suffer more tooth problems because of this. Us desperate dentally phobic people have been known to avoid dentists, struggle on with painkillers, attempt DIY dentistry or worse. In these modern times, it is extremely rare for people to perish from dental conditions, but unfortunately, it can and does still happen if our dental fear gets in the way of our getting much needed help.

Clearly, fixing our fear can be life saving, and is important if it helps us go to the dentist and enjoy better teeth. But is it possible to heal a lifetime of dental anxiety?

This book does not promise to cure our phobias (although this may happen), but it does attempt to help us understand, respect and work with our fears. Often we blame ourselves for our dental phobias and not going to the dentist. We say things like, 'I should have come earlier', and we tell our dentists, 'I must be your worst patient.'

Treatment begins with acknowledging our fears, selecting our support team and reducing our shame. Then, we bravely contact a dentist and make an appointment. Our next right step is to be kind to ourselves. Only then, we pay our dentist a visit, and use additional **Gentle Dental** tricks and techniques to finesse our fear and phobia recovery. Finally, after all this proud progress, we congratulate ourselves, review our adventures, keep up the wonderful work and share the good news. We can do this!

Chapter 3. A better way forward.

What if you are utterly convinced that you and your personal smile sorrows are hopeless, much worse than anyone else's and especially difficult to treat, and that you will never be able to overcome your dental fears and get the help you need? What if you are in so much mental or physical pain, or experiencing such prolonged suffering that you feel like you want to give up?

If this is you, trust me, you are not alone. Do not despair.

If you 'can't bear it any longer', if you feel like 'giving up', 'going to sleep and never waking up again', actively harming yourself or simply somehow neglecting yourself to the point of no return, please think again.

Those of us who experience mental health challenges, and that's an awful lot of us, may feel even worse when confronted by dental problems. Even the most mentally resilient of us may despair in the face of seemingly intractable fear and pain. Warning signs of self harming or suicidal acts include having made threats, pacts, plans or previous attempt(s), recent failure (e.g. in exams, relationships or work), self neglect, a family history of suicide, a perceived or actual loss of concern for others and by others and perhaps, most seriously, a sense of calmness related to having made a decision to commit suicide...

If this is happening to you, DON'T DO IT! There will be more on practicing self care and improving your situation in Chapter 8. Feel free to skip ahead and check it out if you wish.

Or, just for now, until you have finished this book, (by which time you should be feeling a whole lot better), try to imagine me, or someone who cares about you (even if you can't feel their love right now), saying any one or more of the following:

1) 'Tell me about it'
2) 'I hear you'
3) 'You are not alone'
4) 'The part of you that wants to die is the ill part. The part of you wants to live is your well part. Listen to your well part. Help your well part get stronger and your ill part get better.'

5) 'Suicide is messy, painful, difficult ... and dangerous'
6) 'Suicide doesn't fix anything'
7) 'Suicide is final. If you kill yourself, you'll never find out the ending.'
8) 'If you want to kill yourself, imagine calling me, and know that I will say, 'no''
9) 'If you still want to kill yourself, by all means, fine, it's your prerogative... but don't'
10) 'Observe your suicidal thoughts. Then laugh at them and ignore them'
11) 'Breathe'
12) 'Sleep on it'
13) 'Self care is the difference between breakdown or breakthrough'
14) 'Keep taking your prescribed tablets in prescribed amounts'
15) 'Call the Samaritans/ Mind/ your doctor/ therapist/ counsellor/ psychiatrist/ A&E department'
16) 'Carry out a Life Plan instead - let go of your suicidal fantasies and tools, 'phone a friend or help line, and commit to self care one day at a time'.
17) 'It will get better. Your teeth will get better and you will get better.'

If you are reading this and thinking it's not that bad, my teeth and my dental phobia are nowhere near that bad, that's great. Perhaps the suggestion that dental anxiety could lead to suicidal despair even sounds a little melodramatic. But experience tells me that people with dental phobias may experience suicidal thoughts in relation to their teeth, especially when things aren't going so well. On a bad day, it's best to pay attention to any difficult feelings we have and get help.

Even those of us driven to desperation by our teeth can finally find the care we need and go on to lead full, happy and beautifully smiling lives – like Dahlia.

SUICIDE IS NOT AN OPTION

'Dentists kept saying that things were wrong with my teeth and doing loads of things like fillings and extractions. One day I went to the dentist and he took out a tooth, and he looked at the one behind it and said, 'I've just realized that that one's bad as well, and we'll need to take it out too.' Then I realized he'd made a mistake and taken the wrong tooth out first, so I ended up having two teeth out.'

'Is it possible he only saw decay on the other tooth after he'd taken the first one out?' I asked, trying to think the best of this colleague.

Dahlia, a woman in her early forties, shook her head.

'It was the look on his face; he knew he'd done something wrong. Everyone in my family had great teeth, all my cousins, we all noticed teeth. I didn't want to lose any more teeth. I wouldn't have been me without teeth. Even my friend who went to the same dentist said, 'Ooh. You've had a lot of work done', and from that moment on I developed a phobia about losing more teeth.'

'Can you tell me more about that?' I asked.

'My grandmother used to say I had to look after my teeth or I would lose them. I remember when I was little she would take out her false teeth and put them next to her on the dining table while she ate meals. It put the fear of God into me,' Dahlia said.

'Clearly, she had an impact,' I said. 'What was your relationship like with your grandmother?'

'My grandmother didn't like my mum and she didn't like me either because I looked like my mum. She didn't like girls because of things that had happened to her. My grandmother was very dominant. Even my mum was scared of her. Mum did everything my grandmother said and so my mum didn't like me either.'

'I imagine you worried that if you lost more teeth your grandmother and mother would have liked you even less,' I offered.

'Yes,' Dahlia nodded.

'As long as **you** like yourself, I suppose that's the important thing now,' I said.

Dahlia didn't understand this at first so I repeated it.

'Look how well you're looking after yourself these days. You floss, you gave up smoking, you eat better and you come here absolutely religiously,' I reminded her.

'I can't imagine not coming here. It's been almost twenty years now,' Dalia said, nodding.

'What did bring you here in the first place?' I asked.

'I was in tears, literally feeling suicidal, not wanting to lose any more teeth.'

When Dahlia said she was 'literally feeling suicidal', I knew she wasn't exaggerating. She had a fought a long battle with anorexia, depression and anxiety. I remembered times when I liaised with her psychiatrist regarding nutritional advice to keep her teeth healthy without triggering anorexic relapses. We had worked hard to rebuild her smile with crown and bridgework. At one stage her tooth loss phobia was so active she experienced panic attacks with even the slightest and most normal sensations from her teeth and needed regular reassurance. Her panic attacks became more frequent whenever she experienced greater difficulties in her family relationships. Dahlia's care became a combination of dental and mental understanding.

'When I tried you, you were different. You never said bad things to me about my teeth. You were the first dentist I felt safe with. Once I went to a hygienist who said my front teeth were loose. She asked her dentist about it and he didn't know why and said I might lose them and I had a panic attack. You explained about the EDS and I stopped panicking.'

Dahlia had Ehlers Danhlos Syndrome, a condition that made all her ligaments highly elastic and stretchy – including the ones holding her perfectly healthy front teeth into their perfectly healthy gums and sockets.

I had supported Dahlia through the physical and emotional pain caused by her hypermobile joints, fractious family, anorexia and depression. But lately, after much work on her life and herself, Dahlia had triumphed over her circumstances. Her mental and dental health was stable. She had qualified as a nursery nurse, was happily married and (after fertility treatment) blessed with two bright and beautiful daughters. Her youngest daughter had recently started school. Dahlia was considering taking piano and maths lessons with a view to improving herself further.

'What advice would you give to other people wanting to end it all over their teeth?' I asked.

'Don't give up,' Dahlia said.

Dahlia is a nice, wise, gentle and loving lady, and one of my most loyal and long standing clients. So, if you are feeling literally suicidal over your teeth, 'just do what the nice lady says and no one will get hurt' – particularly you. You are worthwhile and important. Please don't give up before the miracle happens.

Chapter 4. Why bother?

Perhaps, by now, you are wondering whether you and your teeth are 'worth all the trouble'? Even though you know it stands to reason that your life would be improved with better dental care enabling you to confidently and comfortably eat, speak, smile, kiss and make love, maybe you are still not sure. Perhaps, like the patient below, you have a worrying symptom that you would prefer not to believe exists.

WHY NOT ME?

I first noticed the lump under my jaw after a brief cold. It involved such a painful episode of earache that I called my doctor to make an appointment, but gave up when I couldn't get an appointment that day.

The lump was on my right, the same side as my earache had been. I assumed it was related, a swollen lymph node or something. In between working, studying, breastfeeding, and parenting a young child, I was very busy. I decided to wait to see if it disappeared, at least a couple of weeks.

The lump did not disappear, but it was painless, and was not getting significantly bigger at any great rate. I decided to visit my doctor none the less, to ask about it.

'It's just a lymph node,' she reassured me.

I went away happy, but chose to keep an eye on it myself. I mentioned it at two further appointments, and each time received the same diagnosis and advice not to worry about it.

By this time the lump had enlarged to the point where I could see the outline of my neck under my jaw had changed. It was more convex on my right side and I could feel it when I pressed the pads of my fingers lightly on the area.

I decided to take independent action. I referred myself to the local hospital oral surgery department. I felt a bit foolish, wasting consultant time with something that was just an enlarged lymph node, but anxiety had me dialling the number for the clinic and making an appointment.

'It's probably just a lymph node,' the consultant said, having taken a full history and palpated the lump inside and outside my mouth.

'Okay,' I said, 'That's a relief.'

'But we'll do a scan, just to be sure,' he added.

Two weeks later, I was back for the follow up appointment. I looked forward to the reassurance that the results of full investigation would give, despite still feeling shame at wasting hospital resources when so many other people had real and greater needs than myself.

'It's a sub mandibular salivary gland tumour, I'm afraid,' my consultant said.

'What?' I asked, shocked and disbelieving. 'I'm a dentist. I refer people to you for these things. I don't have them myself,' I protested.

'When patients ask, 'Why me?'' my consultant responded gently, 'I suggest they consider, 'Why not me?''

Indeed. Two years had elapsed since I had first noticed the lump, and I was only now scheduled to have it removed. I was very conscious of the fact that it was getting slowly bigger.

I went on the internet to research salivary gland tumours and discovered that those in the submandibular region could indeed be malignant. The thought of radiotherapy or chemotherapy in addition to surgery was distressing. My final exams in General Dental Surgery were coming up. My daughter was starting nursery school, and both my parents were ill. I did not need this. I coped by not thinking about it in any deep way and getting on with things, but I found it notably difficult to think ahead to anything after the operation and the biopsy results.

The day after passing my Membership exams, I went into hospital and had the tumour excised along with the gland it was deeply attached to. My recovery was complicated by an allergy to the suture material. I had a four-centimetre scar, some superficial skin numbness, and an asymmetrical neck to show for it.

But the tumour, an unusual myoepithelioma, was benign. Thank goodness. And it had all been removed with the surgery. I felt deeply indebted to my consultant, and lucky and grateful for the serenity that a benign diagnosis offered.

That was eighteen years ago. I have had no recurrence, but I have had an unexpected gift. I am proactive and vigilant about head and neck and mouth cancer screening and referral in my practice. I share my experience with my own clients, particularly when they are going through similar trials.

And if they ask, 'Why me?' I gently suggest they consider, 'Why not me?'

If you are experiencing fear, doubt and denial, rest assured that this is a normal part of making changes in your life. No one can deny that denial is useful. Denial protects us from feeling overwhelmed by experiences until we are more ready to deal with them. Unfortunately, our lovely smiles may be neglected when denial relating to fear of dentists, dental disease, dental diagnoses, dental treatment and yet more dental treatment keeps us from seeking help. Our thoughts and actions around our fears and phobias, which may have kept us safe in the past, may now resist our intentions to grow and be different and hold us back. Choosing to change is an act of courage. Needing and choosing to change does not mean we were foolish in the past, any more than outgrowing our clothes meant we were undersized as children. Personal growth is one of life's gifts and our commitment to it keeps us young and alive in spirit. Later in this book we will learn how to harness this gift to help us in our smile recovery.

Perhaps, for whatever reason, you experience chronic shame and low self esteem around yourself and your smile. (There will be more about combating this in chapter 8.) Just for now, even if you don't think you deserve a healthy, happy, shiny smile, bear with me.

Or perhaps you feel you get along fine, bar the occasional toothache/moment of self consciousness. Perhaps smiling with healthy, happy teeth is vastly overrated, you feel...

But...

Human beings are designed to smile, right from infancy. If for any reason, we can't, won't or don't smile, people are less likely to smile back at us, and we risk living in a world of reflected gloom. Our mouths and eyes form a 'communication triangle' that we look to for information in social interactions with others. If you are covering your mouth with your hand when you smile, smiling without showing your teeth, or if you feel you would smile more often if your teeth looked better, you are at a disadvantage that could affect your self-esteem, relationships and career prospects.

When we smile, we feel better in ourselves, and give a gift to others. When people smile back warmly, returning our gift with interest, it makes us feel even better and even more likely to carry on sharing the love and living a life of ease and connection.

You, just as much as any one else, are 'worth it'. You deserve to enjoy and feel proud of your smile and all that it has to offer and bring to you.

Perhaps you are thinking, 'Why now? I'm not in any pain'. Good news! This is the best time to visit a dentist. When you're not experiencing stressful pain, going to the dentist for preventive care and attention is an excellent idea. 'If it ain't broke, don't fix it' applies to a lot of situations, but in your mouth, where it's hard to see and tell normal from not normal, a regular mouth check is always better than leaving things and worrying or suffering more later. Your dentist, unlike your nearest and dearest perhaps, will tell you if you have bad breath and how to get rid of it, for instance. They will know which patches, lumps and bumps need monitoring, and which need further checking out. And while your dentist is carrying out your smile MOT, they can arrange a spring clean and any other necessary maintenance for your gorgeous teeth and gums.

On the other hand, if you are in pain, perhaps you are thinking, 'If I ignore it, tough it out, it will go away, like it did last time. If I go to the dentist, it will hurt/ make it worse/ they will find other things to do/ they will find something really bad/ etc.' Oh dear. Any pain (or pus, swelling, colour change, ulceration etc.) is a warning sign from our bodies that something is wrong, especially if it lasts, gets worse, keeps coming back, or interferes with our eating, sleeping, talking, working or playing. If, despite your best efforts, you have pain that does not settle down, it is time to seek help from a qualified professional who is trained to put you at your ease, keep you comfortable at all times, provide information and reassurance, and diagnose and treat dental problems. Chapter 6 will help you find the right dentist to help you in your quest.

But perhaps, like many others, you simply can't see the point. 'I've got bad teeth. Everyone in my family has bad teeth/ weak gums/ sensitive teeth/ a sweet tooth/ or some other dental challenge. All my friends/peers/colleagues/ fellow football season ticket holders in the east upper stand etc. have bad teeth. And they manage perfectly well,' you may say. Yes. Maybe they do. For them, in their lives and times. But what if they don't manage, don't have the dental care they need, and just put a brave face on it, literally. What if you never know how they really feel about their dental situation? What if they spend their lives suffering dental pain or are too ashamed to smile showing their teeth? Or, what if they do manage just fine, but you don't. You are allowed to be you, different, wonderful, unique, special and worthy of special care, including special dental care. Dentistry is a constantly evolving profession, with more and more that can be done to improve our looks and our lives, whoever we are and whatever our genes and circumstances.

Or what if, like the patient below, you are still feeling resistant to change, wondering if you can justify the cost of regular or even emergency dental care, and more than just a little annoyed that you are bothered by such concerns in the first place...

BARGAINING

The patient, a fit, middle-aged woman, sat up, and rinsed her mouth.

'Thank you. My teeth feel so much better after you clean them,' she said.

'You're doing well. We'll schedule a maintenance visit for three months time,' her periodontist, a gum specialist, said.

'Do I really need to come every three months?' the patient asked.

'Ideally,' her periodontist said.

'What if I come every six months?' the patient asked.

'There's a risk you will lose more bone around your teeth. Generally, you've already lost a third of the supporting jawbone,' the periodontist said. He pointed to her x-rays, mounted on a light screen.

The patient and her periodontist looked at the x-rays together.

'And you've lost 40% of the bone around your lower incisors,' the periodontist said.

'That's awful,' the patient said. She stared at the incriminating black, white and grey shadows on the x-ray film of her teeth.

The periodontist nodded.

'We'll keep monitoring it,' he said.

'40%,' the patient repeated.

'Yes,' the periodontist said.

'Will I lose my front teeth?' the patient asked.

'Hopefully not,' the periodontist said.

'I thought I was doing so well with my home care,' the patient said.

'It's impossible to clean deep gum pockets, even with electric brushes and interspace gadgets,' the periodontist said helpfully.

'40% is a lot,' the patient said.

'It's better than 50%. Then, the mechanical forces from biting increase the rate of bone loss even further,' the periodontist said.

'I've been flossing since I was 11 years old. It's not fair.'

'It's unlucky. Smoking, pregnancy and diabetes make gum disease worse, but sometimes it's just genetic susceptibility,' the periodontist said.

'I had one miscarriage and a pregnancy, but I never smoked, and I'm not diabetic,' the patient said. 'But both my parents had gum disease.'

'It's just bad luck,' the periodontist said.

'So, when do you want me back? Four months?' the patient asked.

'If we give your teeth a professional clean every three months, that should stop any further bone loss,' the periodontist said.

'It's expensive, inconvenient and time consuming,' the patient said.

'Yes. A bit like going to the hairdresser, except that if you have a bad haircut it grows out,' the periodontist said.

'I know, I know... teeth have to last a lifetime,' the patient said.

'Most people spend more on hair care than dental care,' the periodontist said.

The patient did a quick calculation.

'Guilty. I'm one of them. I surrender,' she said.

She thanked her periodontist, and walked to the reception area.

'I'd like to make an appointment for three months time,' she said.

'Name?' the receptionist asked.

'Dr Kathy Nathan,' the patient said.

Okay, yes, it's me again. If by now, you are wondering whether it is wise to follow the advice of a dentist who is clearly capable of denial and avoidance when it comes to her own dental care, I would hasten to reassure you. I once expressed doubts about my ability to counsel my teenage daughter on keeping herself safe, given my own misspent youth, when a dear friend of mine, a psychotherapist, replied with the immortal words, 'Nuns don't necessarily make the best moral educators.' Sometimes it takes an experienced and largely reformed dental avoider like myself to know and better advise others of us travelling on the road to personal and smile care satisfaction.

Chapter 5. Is dental phobia treatable?

Yes, oh yes. As a dentist with three decades of experience I know that dental phobias and fears are highly manageable conditions. Two main types of dental phobia treatments exist; drugs (general anaesthetics or sedatives) and Cognitive Behavioural methods (managing our thoughts and actions). Both alternatives offer highly dependable phobia solutions. Choosing one or the other in any given situation requires careful consideration. The information below will help, but the final choice is always up to you and your dentist.

Dental phobia treatments:

General Anaesthetic

Some of us are old enough to remember the days when, 'I want to be knocked out,' was the most common request people with dental phobias made. Every year, thousands of people, including many children and maybe yourself, underwent general anaesthetic, or GA, for routine dental care. In 2001, for safety reasons, the General Dental Council restricted the provision of GA's to hospital settings, making it impossible to obtain in general dental practices. Sometimes when a procedure is particularly strenuous, however, a GA is the best and most appropriate choice. You might need major jaw surgery or removal of deeply buried teeth, for example. On these occasions, when truly necessary, general anaesthetic is available by referral to a safe hospital environment, with dedicated equipment and trained staff.

This was the case with Betsy, a woman with a big problem.

A BIG PROBLEM

Betsy's smell greeted me before she did and I knew immediately that her dental problems were serious.

'I'm terrified of you dentists. I know I should have come earlier. I'm in a really bad way. Please tell me you can help me,' Betsy said.

I assured Betsy that she was not alone or at fault for experiencing a healthy disrespect for dentists and dentistry and that I was proud of her for being here now. Together, we looked at her mouth in the clinic. It was not good. Her teeth were loose and rotten, pus drained from her gums and I worried for her health. Tired, pale and ashen in colour, Betsy did not look well.

'I'm so sorry,' I said. 'We can't save them. Your teeth are so decayed and your gums are so poorly, we can't do anything to fix them. Your teeth need to come out for you to get better.'

'Yes, that's what I meant. I want you to take them out. All of them,' Betsy said.

'Oh. Well, yes, of course,' I said.

Betsy was a large, quiet, shy and considerably overweight lady, who had been leading a reclusive life for many years. With little in the way of good nutrition and health care, her teeth were now breaking off, leaving decayed roots sitting in rancid pools of infection in her bright red, bleeding, grossly swollen gums.

'I know I have really bad breath. People turn their heads when I talk to them. If you take all my teeth out, my mouth will get better, won't it? People won't turn away when I talk to them if my gums get better,' Betsy asked.

Sometimes, I reassure people about the freshness of their breath. More often, I encourage people to step up their oral hygiene for the sake and pleasure of enjoying healthy gums and fresher breath. With Betsy, I did neither.

'When you've had all your teeth out, your gums should heal up and your bad breath should disappear,' I said.

'How soon can I have them out?' Betsy asked.

'Well,' I said.

This was the key question. Normally, I would avoid referring clients to hospital for dentistry with general anaesthetic (GA). Many, many times, people asking to 'be knocked out' for dental care succeeded, with a touch of Gentle Dental magic, in having treatment while conscious and going on to enjoy better smiles and self confidence. But sometimes the small but significant added risk of a GA is justified, and Betsy's condition suggested this might be such a case.

'In theory, I could take out all your teeth in four to six visits, over eight weeks or more taking into account recovery time and using local anaesthetic to numb your gums at every visit,' I said, obligingly explaining all possible options.

'I can't bear this any longer,' Betsy said.

'But it's possible, because you're so unwell and you have so many teeth to come out, that the hospital will accept you for a full clearance, as they call it, with general anaesthetic,' I said.

'Yes, please,' Betsy said.

'It's just that I don't know how long the waiting list is. It used to be up to two years for wisdom tooth removal, and I wouldn't want you to be suffering all that time,' I said.

'I really need them out as soon as possible,' Betsy implored.

'Yes,' I said.

I reached for my prescription pad to write Betsy up for antibiotics until active treatment could commence.

'This will hopefully keep the infection from getting worse, while you wait for assessment and treatment,' I said.

'Please,' said Betsy.

'But I want you to call me if things get worse with the infection, in case we need to admit you to hospital as an emergency. And I'll start taking your teeth out myself if we can't get you seen to quickly,' I said.

Betsy nodded, and took the prescription from me. I wrote 'URGENT' in highlighted capitals on her referral letter and posted it first class that day.

One month later, I received a follow up visit from Betsy.

'The hospital were fantastic. I had them all out a week ago with GA and I felt better as soon as I woke up. It must have been all that poison in my body making me feel ill, she said.

I guessed that the oral surgeons, like me, had taken one look at Betsy's mouth and fast tracked her care. Thankfully, Betsy's gums were now healing miraculously and her skin tone looked normal, rosy even. She even reported she was able to eat better now that her mouth was improving, despite being without teeth. Her bad breath was completely gone. We arranged for her to have a first set of false teeth made in another couple of months, once her gums had settled more fully.

'This is for you,' Betsy said shyly before she left. She reached across and placed a small woolen white and lilac teddy bear into the palm of my hand.

'It's beautiful,' I said, cradling its tiny, soft, hand crocheted body.

'I made it for you. Thank you for all you have done for me,' Betsy said.

Sedation

Sedation, another option for those of us with severe phobias, also requires special care and monitoring throughout treatment. Under the influence of relaxant drugs, we are drowsy but conscious while our dental care is carried out. Inhaled or breathed in sedatives such as nitrous oxide ('happy gas') and intravenous (injected) sedatives such as midazolam both require monitoring by a qualified anaesthetist during administration. Oral (swallowed) sedatives such as diazepam are available by prescription from doctors or dentists. All sedatives require a responsible adult chaperone to accompany us to and from appointments safely and to care for us until the effects of the drugs wear off. Often sedatives have the advantage of leaving us with little or no memory of our dental visits and what we have had done. A chaperone can confirm that our dental care did in fact take place according to our wishes!

CUDDLY DUDDLY

Hilary's cracked lower front incisor had a massive abscess, and she was in pain. Her usual dentist had retired, a new dentist did not offer sedation, and I had been recommended.

'I don't want to know anything about it when you work. I'm terrified,' she said.

I believed her, even though many people, even those who have had sedation for years, prefer to manage without when good enough TLC (tender, loving care to you and I), or 'behavioural management', to use the technical term, is available.

But I could tell from Hilary's mouth, scarcely brushed because of a deep, visceral, dislike of oral sensation, that it might take more than skilled techniques, hypnotic suggestion, affirmation and love to ease this part of her dental journey.

We discussed the options. I gave her Lambie, our soft toy, to hold while we talked.

'I don't want him,' she said, handing him back to me.

'Thank you, Lambie, I'll look after you now,' I said, patting Lambie as I rested him on the side board. I briefly worried that I might have offended Hilary with the offer of our most hard working comforter, but decided to move on.

We called Hilary's doctor, son, daughter, husband and denturist to confirm sedative dose, chaperoning, and immediate denture placement. All good.

Hilary was concerned that oral sedation, diazepam, would not be enough to calm her anxiety.

'I've only ever had the needle sedation before. I'm a big woman. Can't I take triple the dose?' she asked.

'You doctor says twice the usual dose is enough,' I said. 'We don't want to cure your dental phobia forever.'

'Okay,' Hilary said, doubtfully. 'My husband's taking the day off work to bring me in. It better work.'

'If it doesn't, we will have to talk again,' I said. 'But I can't take any risks with your health.'

The following week, the 'phone rang. It was Brian, Hilary's husband.

'She took the two tablets half an hour ago, and she says they're not doing a thing,' he said.

I spoke to Hilary, then asked her to pass the 'phone back to Brian.

'She's not aware of an effect, but she's already starting to slur her words,' I said.

By the time Brian arrived, I had to help Hilary out of the passenger seat using a transfer technique I learned from a physiotherapist friend. Hilary was dreamy and legless. I greeted her softly and warmly. We wandered up the ramp to the front door and into the treatment room.

I numbed Hilary's tooth. The adjacent gum was still swollen after a week on antibiotics. I cleaned Hilary's teeth while the anaesthetic took effect. Despite the sedation, Hilary was able to follow instructions to turn her head or rinse her mouth. Finally, I eased the broken tooth out of its infected socket.

'Well done. All finished,' I said, putting a pack over the socket.

'Are you sure?' Hilary asked.

'Very sure. You've done really well. Do you want to see the tooth?' I asked.

'Show Brian,' Hilary said.

Brian was suitably impressed, not the least that Hilary had managed to have the treatment with tablet sedation. Together, we chaperoned Hilary to the car, with her care instructions and follow up appointment confirmed with Brian.

By now, Hilary was much more oriented. It seemed a good time to ask.

'I have a question,' I said.

'Yes?' Hilary asked.

'Where is he from?' I asked, pointing to the small blue penguin Hilary had held throughout her visit.

'He's Cuddly Duddly. I borrowed him from Rosie, my granddaughter,' Hilary said.

'Wow. He's lovely,' I said.

'I thought of him when you gave me Lambie last time,' Hilary said.

'We're never to old to cuddle a soft toy at the dentist,' I agreed.

Cognitive Behavioural Therapy (CBT).

Even if we are fit and well, sedation and general anaesthetic carry additional inconvenience and risks, with potential unwanted side effects such as prolonged drowsiness. For many of us with work to do, machinery to operate or others to care for, the option of sedation is unrealistic –people may depend on our consciousness to do the school run, for example!

Despite the apparent advantages of being 'totally relaxed' or 'put to sleep' for our dental treatment, one of the biggest drawbacks of pharmacological (drug) relaxation methods is that they do little to help with our underlying fears and phobias. In fact, by avoiding our fears, we may even increase both our anxieties and our reliance on chemical methods to manage them.

Many or us find we cope better and ultimately enjoy visits more when we are treated consciously, carefully and lovingly with everything from quality conversation and compassion to hand signals and hypnosis. Cognitive (our thinking) and Behavioural (our actions) Therapy, CBT, is an invaluable addition to simple kindness in helping us overcome our fears. Paying attention to our feelings, thoughts and behaviours gives us the insight, motivation and means to change our whole experience of our dental care and ourselves. CBT is based on well-established and researched techniques for treating anxieties, fears and phobias (referred to interchangeably throughout this book). CBT is one of the cornerstones of the Gentle Dental approach, and will become second nature to you as you put it into practice. Practicing CBT may take a bit more effort to begin with, but will ultimately reap huge rewards.

For those of us who have only ever managed dental care with GA or sedation, using CBT may involve a giant leap of courage and faith. As was the case for Katy, below, our trust may repay us with lasting improvements in our health, appearance and confidence.

BE GOOD

'Be good.'

Her mother's words drifted away as they became separated.

Led into a small room, the girl was told to lie down.

The man seemed big. He had a mask over his face. His eyes looked small behind his glasses.

'Hurry up. Lie down', he said.

She had not met this man before. She did not trust him. She sat up, and got ready to leave.

'Lie down,' he repeated.

'I want to go home,' she said. She struggled.

'Lie still,' he said.

The woman with the man grabbed her arm.

'I want my Mummy,' she cried.

The woman pushed her back down on the bed. The man held a mask over her face.

'Be good and it will be over quickly,' he said.

'Be good...' her mother's words drifted back in her mind just before she lost consciousness.

When the girl awoke, she felt confused, then sick to her stomach. Her mouth was a sea of pain. She vomited. A stream of blood and mucous spurted down her chest and stomach. She cried out. The big man was gone. The woman came back into focus.

'For goodness sake, call if you need the sick bowl,' she said.

'I want my Mummy,' the girl cried.

'Your Mummy will be here in a minute,' the woman said.

But it seemed like ages.

'What happened?' her mother asked when she arrived.

'Lots of children are sick after the anaesthetic,' the woman said.

'Mummy,' the girl sobbed, 'My mouth hurts.'

'That's what you get from eating all those sweeties,' her mother said.

'The operation went very well. We took out all her decayed back teeth and the four rotten teeth at the front,' the woman said.

'I want to go home,' the girl said, reaching out to her mother.

'For heaven's sake, you're six years old. You're a big girl. Stop behaving like a baby,' her mother said.

'Carry me,' the girl implored her mother.

'Stand up. None of the other children behave like this,' her mother said.

She dragged the girl to her feet.

Next time I'll ask your father to come with you. He'll make you behave,' she said...

The little girl, Katy, was now in my practice, on her own, forty years later.

'I don't know why I'm so terrified of the dentist,' she said, 'It took me two years to email your practice. I must have read your website a hundred times before I wrote.'

'Tell me about your experiences with dentists in the past,' I said.

Katy shared her story. And the fact that as an adult she had fallen down a set of narrow stone steps, and cracked several teeth, which were later extracted, again with general anaesthetic. And that she had had such a severe reaction to the anaesthetic that she had been incapacitated with a headache for days and had never gone back to have the remaining roots removed.

'But lots of my friends have been through the same thing, and they've all managed to go to the dentist. I feel awful that I've let my teeth get in such a state.'

'As a child, you were separated from your mother, had extractions with general anaesthetic and suffered nausea, pain, fear and shame. Unlike your friends, you later went through another trauma and yet another general anaesthetic with side effects. Let's not blame the victim,' I said.

We talked. Katy agreed to let me look at her teeth. We introduced raised hand 'Stop!' signals to help Katy manage her fear during her care. To Katy's surprise she managed to have her teeth cleaned at her first appointment.

'They feel different. They look amazing,' she said.

With forty years of staining and calculus gone, they did indeed look different. For the first time I noticed Katy had long dark hair, blue eyes, and was tall and slim.

'You look like Wonder Woman,' I said.

'I feel like Wonder Woman,' Katy said.

Sometimes, when past experience collides with current mishaps, an even greater degree of faith, courage and trust is required. Because all dentists are human (really?!), they (and yes, I include myself) make mistakes. Hopefully not so many or so grave as to completely drain us of our developing confidence, but mistakes that may be off putting nonetheless. When this happens, it may help to keep the big picture in mind – we need our teeth and ourselves to be loved and looked after. A small amount of human imperfection may have to be tolerated and forgiven to achieve this goal. My relationship with Helga is a case in point.

CLUMSY BEGINNINGS

'Hello, Helen,' I said, holding out my hand in greeting.

'It's Helga,' my new client said, shaking my hand.

After apologising for my lateness (stuck in traffic) and getting her name wrong (bad memory), Helga and I got down to business.

'You'll have to use sedation,' Helga said.

'Tell me more,' I said.

Helga had not had dental treatment without sedation for twenty years, since an unfortunate episode involving ineffective local anaesthetic and a prolonged and difficult tooth extraction in her lower jaw. In an unrelated experience, she developed a needle phobia after several juniour staff tried unsuccessfully to take a blood sample, and the woman who later became her favourite phlebotomist left the hospital to work elsewhere.

'Oh, dear,' I said.

Helga agreed I could look at her teeth, as long as I didn't do anything.

I looked at Helga's teeth. I didn't do anything. I explained hand signals, relaxation and breathing techniques. My dental nurse fetched Lambie, our soft toy, for cuddling. For Helga, not me.

I arranged x-rays, and took care of administration. Then I offered Helga a gentle clean.

'Without sedation?' Helga asked.

Her breathing rate had increased. There was fear and tears in her eyes.

'You've managed the checkup so well; I think it would be helpful to try a gentle clean. Our ultrasonic machine is state of the art, a bit like an electric toothbrush and a carwash rolled into one. Any time you put your hand up, we will stop immediately,' I said.

Helga remembered the days of dentistry when dentists scraped teeth clean with sharp metal instruments and dental drills ran on overhead ropes and pulleys. All the equipment was slow, agonizingly slow. But times had changed, and she knew that a better experience of dentistry, without sedation, might help overcome her fear.

'I'll try,' she bravely said.

With Helga's assistance, my nurse and I gently cleaned her teeth, removing decades of accumulated calculus and staining. Throughout, I encouraged Helga to feel Lambie's weight, and breathe slowly and deeply from her stomach, moving Lambie up and down. Every time Helga raised her hand, we stopped for a commercial break. My nurse wiped Helga's mouth; I patted Helga's arm and affirmed her. Helga swallowed, caught her breath, and nodded for us to proceed.

Helga's teeth and gums were very sensitive. I used the lowest of settings on my ultrasonic scaler, and paused regularly. Miraculously, we managed an excellent first pass cleaning.

'That's amazing,' Helga said.

She gazed at her teeth in the mirror, clean for the first time in years.

'Thank you,' she said, tears in her eyes once more.

She reached out and gave me a hug. And my nurse.

'I didn't think I would ever manage treatment without sedation,' she said.

'Thank you for your trust in me,' I said.

'My family will be amazed,' she said.

Despite my clumsy beginning with Helga, and her painful and clumsy experiences with previous health carers, Helga, a brave and forgiving woman, had tried again, and triumphed over her fear.

'You are a champion,' I said.

If you have read this far, and if like Katy, Helga and many, many others, making the effort to improve your smile now seems worthwhile and maybe even achievable, even if only a little bit, you are ready to consider your very own Gentle Dental **SMILE!** plan. Well done!

PART TWO

YOUR PERSONAL **SMILE!** PLAN

Having discovered or accepted that you are indeed the wonderful owner of a dental fear or phobia and become ready to secure some sensational soothing smile care, it is time to read on. Even if you are not ready, Part Two will help you become ready and give you the information you need to make better choices about your dental care. It will help you achieve healing physically, mentally and dentally, just by remembering to **SMILE!**

SMILE! is our very own handy Gentle Dental memory prompt to help you follow 'Five Simple Steps to Smiling Success'. By remembering to **SMILE!** you will:

Select your support team and dentist.

Make an appointment.

Indulge in self-care.

Lift off!

And

Enjoy!

Chapter 6.

Step One:

Select your smile supporters

Choose your support team

Facing dental fear begins with telling others about our fears and being out and proud about our anxieties and phobias. Sharing with people we trust helps us to feel connected and hopeful. Supportive pals are a powerful shame and fear-busting tool.

In our mission to turn **FEAR**, our '**F****k **E**verything **A**nd **R**un' instincts, into '**F**ace **E**verything **A**nd **R**ecover' triumphs, we have potentially powerful allies. These are the supportive friends, lovers, partners, family, colleagues, neighbours, carers, priests, doctors, strangers on a train, and anyone, anywhere, who will listen to our experiences, thoughts and feelings with compassion, empathy and understanding. Even our pets, plants or soft toys will do, as long as we feel heard and loved.

Many Gentle Dental clients bring very special people with them to share their experience. Having someone you trust literally or metaphorically hold your hand might be all you need to help you cross the threshold of a new dental practice and move toward a better life. Think about whether you would like your chaperone to come with you into the treatment areas (with your dentist's blessing) or simply just be there for you in the lounge room while you receive care.

Ideally, friends and family are welcome in the treatment room if the person receiving dental care wishes – that would be you! Holding hands, receiving gentle shoulder pats, music of your choice, soft toys (for young and old!), rest breaks and magic numbing jelly before effective local anaesthetic (the 'sleepy juice') are all great additions to good, basic dental care. Many of us feel reassured by being told what's happening and watching while our smiles are attended to. Some of us don't, and that's okay too. Your supporters, who are sometimes also your dental caregivers, will ideally be there to listen to you and meet your needs.

Ila, below, brought her mum with her on her visits in addition to enjoying the comforts of our most loving and hardworking soft toy, Lambie.

HAVE YOU GOT THE LAMB?

'Hello Gentle Dentist Harrow

I am 36 years old and haven't been to the dentist for years (apart for a professional clean about 3 years ago) because I am so scared going to the dentist! I have had toothache on and off for about 3 months – it's got so painful I can't eat anything without it kicking in and now I can't brush that side of my mouth.

I have been paying dental insurance for the past 3 – 4 years hoping it would get me to the dentist – but it never.'

I read Ila's email, and was reminded of people who join a gym hoping to get fit, and then never use their membership. For better or for worse, Ila's pain had now prompted action. I emailed back, and Ila arrived at Gentle Dental with her mother that same week.

After a warm welcome, Ila and her mother, Carly, accompanied me to the treatment room. Ila, a tall, classically leggy blonde with tumbling hair and rock chick boots, jeans and t-shirt, unfolded herself into the dental chair. At 37years of age, she held a lot of responsibility in her role as property manager for a sheltered housing association. Now it was her turn to be looked after.

Ila had gone quiet, with a wide, startled look on her face.

'Lambie,' I said to my nurse, who passed Ila our soft cuddly toy. I invited Ila to hold lambie on her tummy and feel his comforting weight going up and down as she breathed.

'Mum?' I said to Carly, inviting her to pull up her chair to the head of the dental setting.

With myself on Ila's right, my nurse on her left, Lambie on her tummy, and her mother cradling her head and stroking her hair and forehead, we formed a little nest.

Between charting Ila's teeth, passing bibs, safety glasses, tissues, mirror, and anaesthetic, my nurse held Ila's hand and gently cheered her on.

With support, encouragement and her own considerable courage, Ila had her first, most troublesome tooth out. She placed her 'I'm a star' sticker proudly on the lapel of her biker jacket as she left with Carly.

On her second appointment, Ila started her visit with the question, 'Have you got the lamb?'

Over the next four visits, Ila had seven white fillings, and several more badly broken down tooth roots and a wisdom tooth removed, all with love, local anaesthetic, and our little nest.

Later, a flurry of emails ensued when it transpired that the insurance company had sent her claim forms to a neighbouring colleague, but eventually these were collected, completed, copied, collated and submitted. Finally, Ila recouped some of her dental insurance subscription value.

Barely a week later, I received a big, bright, glittering thank you card in the post.

'Dear Kathy,

I just wanted to say thank you for making my mouth healthy again after avoiding the dentist for 24 years! And a HUGE thank you for all your patience and for giving me the confidence to start going to the dentist again – I wish I found you years ago! See you in 3 months!

With love Ila x

> P.S. A special thanks to Lambie too – a very special lamb!!!'

'What? Hold a lamb?' I hear you say. Yes. No matter how old we are on the outside, when we are feeling fear, we can be very little on the inside. But I do acknowledge that sadly, personal, cultural and gender restraints might stop us from bringing our mums, dads and cuddly toys to the dentist. If you, like Ron, below, prefer to keep your vulnerabilities private, there are still options for support, including telephone contact with understanding friends and, of course, the dental team itself.

> WALK TALL
>
> Ron lay at the foot of the stairs, curled up into a foetal position, crying.
>
> 'I can't do it,' he said.
>
> 'You won't be doing it alone,' I said.
>
> I patted his arm lightly.
>
> 'Is there someone we can call for you? Someone who knows you're here today?' I asked.
>
> 'My mate, Brian, he knows I'm here,' Ron said.
>
> 'Let's give him a call,' I said.
>
> I sat just next to Ron, at the foot of the stairs. Ron called Brian.
>
> 'I don't know how I'm going to do it,' he said.

I could hear Brian's encouraging noises from the other end of the line.

Ron hung up.

'We'll do it together,' I said, walking with Ron to the treatment room.

Ron sat in the dental chair.

I struggled to adjust the headrest. Ron was quite a bit taller than my 5'6", and I had to reach up to get the chair comfortable for him.

'How tall are you, Ron?' I asked.

'5'4",' Ron replied.

'On a good day?' I asked.

'6'1",' Ron said.

We numbed up Ron's gum and tooth, with copious hand holding and anaesthetic jelly and liquid. Ron and I chatted while the anaesthetic took effect. He came for treatment regularly - about once every five years. We had a lot to catch up on.

'When I was last here, you took out my two smashed up lower teeth, remember. The ones that got broken when I was playing against Milwall for QPR,' Ron reminded me.

'How could I forget,' I said.

Ron, an ex-professional footballer, was defending when the injury happened. I was actually relieved when knee injuries forced him into a change of career. As a plumber, he worked hard, but never suffered similar traumas.

Now Ron had a decayed and cracked wisdom tooth wobbling around in his mouth. With continual calming conversation, we gently delivered the tooth from its socket.

'Is it done?' Ron asked in amazement as I showed him the gauze pack he would need to bite on for half an hour to protect the developing clot.

'All done,' I said.

'Do you want to have a look at the tooth?' I asked.

I offered him the sad specimen, wrapped in tissue.

'I don't want to see it,' Ron said.

'Sure. We'll dispose of it thoughtfully,' I said. 'You won't miss it.'

'I know. I knew I had to get it out ages ago. I worked up my nerve to come back, and then you where shut for a while.'

'We were closed for refurbishment. How come you didn't go somewhere else?' I asked.

'I hate dentists, but I love you,' Ron said.

'I know. It's not personal. I'm the dentist people love to hate,' I said.

'That's it exactly,' Ron said.

He promised to make another appointment, just as soon as his work got less busy.

'Call any time. You're always in my mind,' I said.

'Will do,' Ron said.

> He left Gentle Dental smiling, off to his next job, walking ten feet tall.

However, whoever, whenever, wherever, the love of supportive people and objects may be the magic balm we need to get us to our dentist when our overworked will power is exhausted. Our next challenge, then, is to find the right dentist to visit for when we, and our support team, are ready.

Choose your dentist

Ideally, you will be able to search and select a dentist who will understand, respect and accommodate your specific, wonderful, special needs. The right dentist will help you overcome your phobias and feel good about yourself - and your beautiful smile. Begin by making your very own Ideal Dentist Wish List and sharing it with your support team who will hopefully help you in your quest. You may want to consider the following as you begin your search:

You might want your ideal dentist to be...

Affable: kind, loving, approachable, recommended, tried and trusted, with a reassuring website or printed information and friendly, caring staff. 'Word of mouth' (no pun intended!) recommendations are really useful, as are websites where you can research a dental practice before you visit. Website testimonials are the next best thing to personal recommendations.

Available: local and/or easily accessible, willing to be contacted by 'phone, letter, email, online or in person and open hours and days convenient to your schedule.

Able: All dentists should be registered with the General Dental Council and their practices inspected by the Care Quality Commission. If you are at all unsure, this can be checked online. An ideal dentist is also experienced in special care dentistry, willing to offer longer appointment times and working in suitably well equipped, relaxing, comfortable premises.

Affordable: It might seem strange to place fees last on the list of potential ideal dentist attributes, but the qualities of kindness, availability and ability are almost certainly remembered long after price is forgotten. Having both given and received NHS and private dental care, I can attest to the benefits of investing time and money to achieve results. In the UK, an ideal dentist is often found in private practice. If you don't have the means for private care, there are several options. You could select an NHS dentist who meets almost all your requirements, you could request referral to a specialist (and there may be a waiting list for this), or you could beg, borrow (please don't steal!) or save the funds you need to see the dentist you prefer privately. Some people forgo a holiday, which might last a week or two, to invest in their smiles, which last a lifetime. Another common way many people save, which also improves their health, is by giving up smoking. Others compare the cost of their annual investment in hair, nail or beauty treatments and decide to give their teeth top billing as well. Whatever you decide, make it a positive choice and be proud of your decision.

Having thought it over, you might extend your research by dropping into dental practices you are interested in, making telephone contact or looking at virtual shop fronts online before you make a commitment.

Perhaps, as Leila discovered through the magic of social media, you already know a good enough dentist willing and able to help you out in an hour of need.

A FACEBOOK REFERRAL

'I'm so scared! It's the first time I've admitted this to anyone but I've not been to a dentist for over 20 years, I'm just petrified! Literally. I fell over last night and broke my 2 front teeth really badly. I have to confront my fear now. Oh god, this is huge for me. Can you help me?' the facebook message read.

My friend, Leila, had woken up on a sofa bed in the flat of her drinking buddy from the night before. A large part of her two front teeth were missing. Leila was in shock. She contacted Stuart, my sweetheart and social networking maestro, who referred Leila to me for advice.

'Leila, my love, so sorry to hear of your news. Not going to the dentist for 20 years due to fear is very common (trust me, you have some excellent company), but breaking front teeth is distressing. There are many things that can be done. First things first... Are you okay otherwise? Any broken bones, etc? You will need to see the doctor/A&E if so. Next... Are you in pain? Soft diet and painkillers (paracetamol) are advised... Next... Are you up to date with your tetanus vaccinations? Back to GP if needed... Now... You will need to see a lovely dentist...' I replied.

The first thing I did when Leila came through the door was to give her a big, loving, therapeutic hug. She burst into tears.

'Well done for getting here,' I said.

With Leila crying on and off, we all trooped into the care room.

Despite twenty years of fear, shame, and now, two traumatized front teeth, Leila's mouth was in reasonable condition.

'Your teeth and gums are generally fine,' I immediately affirmed.

'I was so scared they were all falling out,' Leila said.

We talked about her mild acid erosion and tooth brushing abrasion and how to protect her smile from further enamel loss.

At last, Leila began to relax. I looked at her cracked upper central incisors.

'How did the accident happen?' I asked.

'I don't remember,' Leila said.

Leila was covered in bruises on the right side of her body, but could not recollect the fall that was the likely cause of all her injuries. It was not the first time she had experienced a blackout after a night of drinking, but it was the first to result in such devastating injury.

We talked about alcohol – it's impact on her health, her current habits, total intake, and the suggested safe limits. Given past experience in simply 'cutting down', Leila decided, with reservations regarding the effects on her social life, to quit drinking. I acknowledged her choice and gave her information on support groups should she need it.

Then, while Leila held the mirror and cradled Lambie, our soft toy, I restored her teeth.

At intervals my dental nurse patted Leila's arm and asked if she was okay.

Leila nodded.

Her fractures, despite their size, had not injured the nerves of her teeth. One big spring clean and two white fillings later, with no injections or drilling needed, Leila's smile was fixed.

Now Leila could not stop smiling.

When I contacted her later that week, she was still smiling, very relieved, and very grateful.

A short while later, I received a message, via facebook, of course, that said it all;

'Hi Stuart and Kathy,

I just wanted to send you both a big *thank you* for your loving care & attention over the past few days, it has been just wonderful.

You were totally amazing, so professional & you put me at ease right from the start with your care & love. You are such a natural at your job & you made it so easy for me, and believe me it really was my biggest fear. WOW! I cannot thank you enough.

With lots of love,

Leila xxx'

Maybe, like Leila, you have a wide social network that includes a dentist you can trust. Maybe you are comfortable using social media to find a dentist you trust by asking your online and connected friends, family, colleagues and associates. But if not, no problem. There is always the option of typing your way to a groovy new dentist using the wonders of the world wide web. When googling, there are some key words, phrases and questions you can use to refine your search for the 'right one'. The terms 'nervous', 'fearful', 'anxious', or 'phobic' in front of 'dental patient' can all give your search engine extra clues to help find your ideal dentist.

If you are new to an area or don't know who to ask, the direct approach can work just as well when calling or visiting a potential new dentist. Asking, 'Do you look after nervous dental patients?' might be all you need to say to a busy receptionist to get the extra information and reassurance required to move on to the next step in your **SMILE!** Plan.

If you have additional needs as well as your fabulous phobia, try asking, 'Do you do Special Care Dentistry?' This is the branch of dentistry that helps make dental care more accessible for all of us, whether we are simply phobic, neurologically challenged, wheelchair abled or have any other interesting special needs. Asking to have your particular needs met is good self care and will help you decide if a dentist is right for you.

The experiences of the following people may inspire you to seek dental care yourself. Where others have travelled, so might you, with the security and support you deserve.

ASPIRING TO ASPERGER'S

I like to think I enjoy a few autistic traits myself, as do many of us probably - it is a spectrum phenomenon after all. But I knew something was even more special about Malcolm from the day I met him. He arrived for his appointment wearing a dark, crumpled and worn suit with an unironed shirt and stained tie. His shoes were unpolished and he spent most of the time looking down at them as he shuffled into the clinic.

'Hello, Malcolm,' I said, on his most recent visit.

'Hello, Dr Nathan,' he replied, in a thin, high voice.

'How are you? Any recent changes to your health or your life,' I asked.

'My health is the same as ever, but do you know what that council is planning to do now?' Malcolm challenged me.

'Oh, dear,' I said. 'It doesn't sound good.'

Over the twenty or so years I had been looking after Malcolm's teeth, Malcolm had been updating me on the inner workings of his neighbouring council's planning committee decisions. He had regularly attended all their meetings until on one occasion, presumably exhausted by his adversarial questions of their every proposal, they had barred him from further visits. Now he followed their fortunes through newspapers and websites. Why he didn't prefer to monitor the progress of his more local council's work, I never ascertained.

'Do come through,' I said.

Together, Malcolm, my nurse and I attended to his teeth. Malcolm had a habit of wincing in response to bright lights, noisy drills and strange smells, touches or tastes, a sign that he was experiencing sensory overload. I offered him our safety sunglasses before turning on the overhead light and maintained a calm, quiet approach with a gentle minimum of handling.

'I'm just going to give your teeth a little polish,' I said, showing Malcolm the polishing paste on its tiny rubber cup in its dental handpiece.

Malcolm opened his mouth obligingly and we carried on. Using the 'tell, show, do' approach, I continued to prepare Malcolm for his care, explaining and demonstrating each stage in advance. Over the years, the practice environment and visiting ritual had varied slightly, but wherever possible with this comforting element of preparation.

'All done,' I said.

'They're considering granting permission for the historic building at the top of the park to be converted into a public house and allowing the duck pond to be converted into a car park,' Malcolm said.

It would be great if the council looked after its parks and buildings as well as you look after your teeth,' I said.

'My teeth are doing well, aren't they?' Malcolm agreed.

'Yes, they are,' I said. 'And so are you.'

Malcolm's love of consistency ensured he attended for all his dental appointments, without fail. As I do for all clients, irrespective of age, gender or position on the autistic spectrum, I presented Malcolm with his 'Well Done' sticker for being good at the dentist.

'Thank you,' said Malcolm, momentarily looking up.

He peeled the plastic backing off the sticker and affixed it to his suit jacket lapel, on the very same suit he had been wearing at every one of his visits for the last two decades. He looked fabulous.

SHOUTING AT ISAAC

It is not my usual habit to shout at my clients. But 84-year-old Isaac was very hard of hearing, and shouting seemed to help.

Isaac was referred to Gentle Dental by the dental laboratory I use for denture additions and repairs. After a fall, two of his teeth were very loose.

'How did you fall?' I asked.

'What?' Isaac asked.

I removed my facemask and turned to Isaac so he could lip-read, if that helped.

'How did you fall?' I enunciated clearly.

'What?' Isaac asked.

'How did you fall?' I shouted.

'I fell on the edge of a carpet in the lounge,' Isaac said.

I checked Isaac over.

'Your nose has been bleeding, and it's a bit crooked. It might be broken,' I said.

'It's fine,' Isaac said.

'Have you had any other falls recently,' I asked.

'Just one, a month ago,' Isaac said.

'I'll write you a letter to take to Accident and Emergency,' I said.

'No, no doctors. I hate doctors,' Isaac said.

I continued shouting at Isaac while I numbed up his teeth, took impressions of his mouth and denture, and took the two extremely loose teeth out.

Later, I showed Isaac how to use his denture with the new teeth added. The denture, decades old, fitted only where it touched. I demonstrated the use of a fixative gel for Isaac.

'I have a bad memory,' Isaac said.

'The instructions on how to use the glue and look after your false teeth are written down,' I shouted, pointing at the box with the denture care samples.

Isaac nodded, paid for his care, and slowly made his way to the waiting car.

I instructed his driver to take him straight to A&E to have him checked over more thoroughly.

When the 'phone rang the next morning, my nurse handed it to me.

'You need to come over and help me,' Isaac said.

'Are you okay, Isaac? What seems to be the problem?' I shouted down the 'phone, worried.

'My denture is loose,' Isaac said.

I explained I wouldn't be able to do a home visit, but I held the line while Isaac fetched the box of samples we had given him.

'Remember, you need to use glue with the denture,' I shouted.

'Oh, yes,' Isaac said.

I talked Isaac through finding the adhesive, unscrewing the lid, squeezing out a pea sized amount at three separate points on the fitting surface of the denture, ('the side without teeth, Isaac,') and putting the denture in his mouth.

'How is that now?' I shouted down the 'phone.

'It's fine,' Isaac said.

The next day, Isaac rang again.

'Can I use mouthwash?' he asked.

'Yes, it's okay now,' my nurse shouted as loudly as she could.

The day after, Isaac called again.

'Where can I find this glue?' he asked.

'The supermarket and pharmacies,' I shouted.

> 'Can I call you again if I need to?' Isaac asked.
>
> 'Any time,' I shouted.
>
> Isaac never did go to Accident and Emergency, having instructed his driver to take him straight home. He did not consent to me calling his doctor. I was comforted in the knowledge that he lived with his wife and adult son, who I imagined would keep an eye on him. And when he didn't call the following day, I missed caring for him, and shouting at him.

If you are even slightly tempted to think of yourself as a 'burden' or a 'nuisance', I beg you to think again. Caring for those of us with special needs is one of the most rewarding branches of dentistry there is. Every time I work with someone to overcome their challenges and win a better smile, I am gifted with the satisfaction of professional achievement and more importantly perhaps, a real sense of connection with my clients. Go on. Give your chosen dentist an opportunity to share the love that is there for you - which is what our next chapter is all about.

Chapter 7.

Make an appointment.

The 'M' in our lovely Gentle Dental **SMILE!** mnemonic launches us yet closer to our gorgeous grinning goal with our next call to action. It commits us to a dental visit by making an appointment. In case this seems overwhelming, perhaps focusing on this action in two parts is helpful, first by making a decision to trust, and then, by taking a leap of faith.

A decision to trust:

Prolonged vigilance and avoidance of dental care is stressful and counter productive, making our dental anxieties and our fear of the dentist even worse. Often, our dental distrust has lead to worsening problems, pain and suffering. If we could fix our dental problems by ourselves, us phobics would, and many of us try.

Acknowledging our need for professional dental help is a brave step in our smile recovery. It requires sufficient humility to accept that we can't do this dental thing on our own, even if we have been trying to for a long time, and even if we have managed sort of okay in the past.

Now we are called to gather courage (our own or our supporter's) and make contact with the very object of our fear – the dentist. But first, we might take a moment to make a conscious decision to trust our dentist and the dental process we are about to commit to. We do this by reassuring our inner child, the part of us that is most likely to be the source of our fear.

Imagine that there is a small, scared child with toothache that you are taking to the dentist. What will you say to this child (without using the words like 'hurt' or 'pain' that might make things worse!) to enable them to trust you and to keep them safe, comfortable and well?

Using your own positive, soothing phrases, or the examples below, try saying aloud something along the lines of the following:

'The dentist will make your teeth all better so you can smile again.'

'I will be with you the whole time.'

'I will make sure you are in safe hands.'

'If you need a break to cough or swallow, or anything else, just raise your hand and the dentist will stop.'

'When your teeth are all fixed, I will get you a prize!'

Now say these phrases again with love and affirmation to your very own inner child.

As with all promises to small children, it is vital that we follow through in order to maintain trust and credibility. Our precious inner children are no exception to this rule. If we have been thorough in researching and selecting the right dentist, this shouldn't be too difficult. A prize at the end of a dental visit can be anything from a hug from a friend or a trip to the library to a designer handbag, an overseas holiday staying in a five star hotel, or more. The successful achievement of your shiny new smile might be your greatest gift to yourself of all, and all that you need and want to feel rewarded. Whatever you can afford and desire, provided it's healthy, safe, legal and kind, you have my blessing to indulge. Use your imagination!

A leap of faith:

At this point, when committing to action, many of us proudly phobic people may be forgiven for thinking, 'I can't do this.' Contacting a dentist, or saying 'yes' to treatment, is usually well out of our comfort zone, or at the very least, unfamiliar, particularly if we have tried and failed before (I prefer to think of these as warm-up attempts or learning experiences).

Fortunately for our **SMILE!** progress, there is another way forward. The most useful and appropriate question we can ask ourselves is, 'How will I do this?'

And the answer is 'Not alone.'

Now is a great time to call on your support team for help. If you are too frightened at this stage to go it alone, one of your supporters can email, book online, or make the call for you, preferably with you having advised them in advance of your availability, or in shouting distance so they can confirm a convenient time and day.

Or, you could call the dentist with your supporter nearby, or after telling them you're about to. Or you could book online or email the dentist/dental clinic of your choice to get the ball rolling if picking up the phone feels like too much at this stage.

A LEAP OF FAITH

'I can't do it today. I just can't. I don't feel well enough,' Nick said.

Nick, a gifted fine artist in his late thirties, had cancelled his appointment for the extraction of a massively infected wisdom tooth at very short notice.

'Do you mean you don't feel well enough mentally, or physically?' I asked.

'I can't get my head around it,' Nick replied. 'I keep worrying about what might happen if something goes wrong.'

Nick had coped very well with his first visit the previous week, and had been delighted with the change in his mouth after his scaling and polishing hygiene treatment, his first for some time. He had seemed quite keen to have the tooth in question removed. It had been draining pus out of his gum and leaving a bad taste in his mouth for years.

Legal advisors tell dentists never to hide or underestimate potential complications of dental procedures, and to ensure informed consent has been properly obtained. Nick had been thoroughly briefed on the alternatives to his proposed extraction, the benefits and disadvantages of each option, and the aftercare he would require. Untoward events that might arise during or after the removal of the tooth had been explained. Nick had authorized a written consent form, complete with the proposed treatment plan, information and disclaimers, for his record.

The image of Nick's tooth on the full mouth x-ray, a molar sitting in a bed of pus, his surrounding jawbone eaten away by infection, flashed through my mind. Somehow, I felt it would be unhelpful to remind Nick of the real and potential ill consequences of leaving the tooth in place, compared to the tiny risk of complications from its extraction.

'You don't have to have it done today,' I said, 'But I am looking forward to helping you with it as soon as possible.'

'You know how it is, with everything that's been happening with my family, I just don't feel like I could cope with it right now.'

Nick was not in contact with his parents, and had recently fallen out with his only sister after her less than credible husband had denied damaging one of Nick's paintings.

'You're feeling quite alone right now,' I said.

'Exactly. This is a difficult time for me,' Nick said. 'I don't like my house, and I know I'll feel depressed as soon as I come home after the appointment, when I'm on my own.'

'Is there anyone besides your family who would be able to come with you and take you home?' I asked.

'I have friends I can call before and after, but no-one right here. And I haven't even got the right food in the house,' Nick said.

'How would it be if you spoke to your friends before and after the visit, and we made sure you had some food to take home? And we'll call you to make sure you get home,' I said.

'I think I will be okay, I do have some food here, but a call afterwards would be great,' Nick said.

We confirmed Nick's appointment for that afternoon.

When Nick arrived, he was much more positive, having had a good breakfast and phoned his friends. The troublesome tooth was delivered safely, comfortably, and uneventfully.

My dental nurse presented Nick with a complimentary tin of soup she had brought from her own home, to help him feel nourished, in every sense of the word. Nick started crying.

'I went to three or four dentists, trying to find the right one. You were the only ones I felt I could trust to take that tooth out,' he said.

When I rang Nick an hour later, he was in his car, had phoned a friend, and was on his way to stay with another friend who would feed and care for him until he felt stronger. He was feeling fine.

A week later, I spoke to Nick again. His tooth socket and spirits were much improved. We talked about his home life. About how it might be better for him to be less isolated domestically. And about how his caring post operative companion, Julia, seemed much more than just a good friend.

'She does want to be with me, but I don't feel it's fair to ask her to be in a relationship with me because of my depression and anxiety,' Nick said.

'True,' I agreed. 'But everyone comes with baggage, and good relationships tend to have a protective effect on mental health.'

I shared my own experience of how much better I felt when in the shelter of loving others.

'You know, I did think this whole tooth business was the worst thing that could have happened to me. But now I see it's got me out of my house and together with Julia, who knows, maybe for the long term,' Nick said.

Nick added that his whole mouth was feeling much better. He said he was popping home that day to pick up his post, and returning to Julia's afterward.

Not everyone finds love in the aftermath of making a dental appointment and having their teeth attended to. And not everyone has friends available to care for them during normal working hours or outside business hours when they are tied up with family and other commitments.

That's okay. That's what answering machines, voicemail and social media are for. Just leave a message, post, tweet, or do whatever you must to get your voice out there, to declare that you are going to call your dentist for an appointment. This public declaration of commitment will massively improve the odds of your following through, all on behalf of your lovely happy smile, and all in your favour. Then, when you have honoured your intention, call, post, tweet, shout out, or whatever, and tell the world, your best friends and their neighbours that you have done it. Feel proud.

'But what if I really am all alone, with only my black Labrador, furry feline friends, cosy cuddly toys, flat screen TV, etc., for company,' I hear you ask.

This too is not a problem. Sharing your intentions and triumphs with your preferred pets, faithful toys and/or beloved objects and icons is absolutely okay.

'I don't have pets or soft toys, and I don't talk to my TV. Or my potted plants,' I hear you protest.

Okay, then. Now is the time to bring out the heavy artillery.

The Spiritual Approach

Most of the advice and suggestions in this book are based on sound well-tested principles in the practice and psychology of special care dentistry. These next are not. But they are worth a try.

If you are currently isolated, you may still choose not to be alone, spiritually speaking. A spiritual answer, if you are willing to try it, might be for you. Using prayer, calling your intentions in to the universe, writing down your goals and posting them in your 'God box', lighting a candle in dedication to your cause, planting a tree in honour of your plan, opening to the possibility in your mind, making a charitable donation to a worthy cause to affirm your decision, meditating on the action beforehand, and so forth, will all work if you let them. It is the decision to invest in a power greater than yourself, a higher power, if you like, that is important here.

'This is all new age bullsh*t,' I hear you say.

Work with me. Please. It might seem naïve, intangible and backward, but then how has rational thinking and any other method you have tried so far helped you? If, like many other still suffering dentally phobic people, you are feeling alone, scared and avoidant, a spiritual answer might be your best bet. You have nothing to lose other than your (quite understandable) cynicism, fear, shame and false pride.

Tell you what. You don't even have to believe in it. You only have to try it. Think of it as a faith experiment. I promise you I won't tell anyone. If you're feeling even in the slightest bit foolish, rest assured that your secret is safe with me. All you need to do is call upon something other than yourself to give you the strength you need to make an appointment with your dentist and see how it works. After all, your best thinking so far has brought you to your current state and no further. If you want to keep getting what you're getting, keep doing what you're doing, as the saying goes. Doing something differently might be the answer. So try it.

Simply practise your own personal ritual of faith and then…

DO IT!

Yes. Call your dentist. While you are full of hope, intention, connectedness, love, peace and serenity. Call your dentist. Make an appointment. Remembering that 'action is the magic word', or, as some people have been known to put it, 'faith without works is dead'. Call your dentist.

Then celebrate! Practise gratitude, if you feel so moved, for your newfound courage and flex your fabulous spiritual muscles even further by giving thanks in the same way you invoked your personal higher power beforehand. It's all good/God, whatever you choose to call it, however you choose to use it, and however you choose to attribute your success and give thanks because of it.

So now, by the grace of yourself/ your inner child and caring adult/ your social network/ God/ whoever and whatever, you have contacted your dentist of choice and made an appointment.

Well done. It is time to put your feet up and relax. Well, partly. Along with several other tips and tricks to get you in great shape for the next stage of your smile care adventure, our next chapter is all about self care.

Chapter 8.

Indulge in self-care.

The 'I' in **SMILE!** reminds us to ready ourselves for dental care by first and foremost putting our own personal care plan into action.

Indulgence is not an indulgence when it comes to improving our health. Self care is not selfish. Self care is often the difference between break down and break through when we are making courageous changes in our lives. Indulgence, self care, pampering, personal health management or however we refer to it, it is an essential part of overcoming our fears and phobias and a way to strengthen ourselves for the changes ahead.

Prepare for your dental visit with excellent self-care.

GENERAL WELLBEING

The first part of our phobia fighting preparation involves getting our general health in order. Everyone from our mothers to the government would be delighted if we just followed a few simple guidelines to improve our wellbeing:

1. Keep our weight in healthy limits.
2. Eat well – more fruit, vegetables and wholegrains and less salt, saturated fat and refined sugars.
3. Drink sensibly.
4. Quit smoking.
5. Stay active.
6. Improve our sleep.
7. Attend to our sexual health.
8. Take up cancer screening opportunities.
9. Get all our vaccinations.
10. Practice safe sun – avoid prolonged, intense exposure to sunshine.
11. Take our prescribed medications and avoid non-prescription drugs.

The first two items on the general wellbeing checklist above deal with how we nourish ourselves. We all know that sugar, sadly, causes tooth decay, but in case you were wondering how else diet relates to dental health, think about the old time sailors whose teeth fell out from scurvy, a vitamin C deficiency due to lack of fresh fruit and vegetables on long voyages. Are you getting your five servings a day? Even obesity is being linked to gum disease because fat creates inflammation in our bodies - yet another reason to eat well and stay active.

Items 3, 4 and 11 deal with non-food substances we may put into our precious bodies. This is obviously of major relevance to our general heath, but in the context of our **SMILE!** program, I will share some specific reflections and recommendations regarding smoking, drinking and drugs, and the considerable impact these have on our lovely smiles.

SMOKING CESSATION

Tobacco causes mouth cancer, tooth discolouration, decay, bad breath and gum disease. Whether it is your first attempt to stop smoking (like Heather and Gianni, below), or whether you have tried many times before, do not give up on giving up. New methods to support you are constantly being developed, and the more quit attempts you make, the more likely you are to stay smoke free as you learn more about what triggers relapse and how to manage. Go for it!

JEDI MIND MELT

Heather, a photographic stylist, was facing an awkward dental challenge in her life, and in her image conscious industry. At the age of sixty, her teeth were falling out.

'Please, I don't want to lose all my teeth,' Heather said.

'You do have serious gum disease,' I said. 'but if we clean your teeth and you're able to give up smoking, we might be able to stop it from going any further.'

Heather's brow furrowed.

'Have you thought about giving up smoking?' I asked.

'Oh, it's a horrible habit, I know I should,' Heather said.

'Have you tried giving up before?' I asked.

'No, never,' Heather said.

'One in five people who give up for twenty four hours never smoke again,' I began, sharing the facts and figures of smoking cessation.

I gave Heather a Smokefree booklet to support her first quit attempt, with further encouraging affirmations. Then, after a thorough clean of her smile, we talked about the finer points of oral hygiene.

'I do love a good gadget, I do,' Heather said, coming to grips with floss and interdental bottle brushes with impressive speed.

'You have fantastic dexterity. You are my best new flosser this week,' I said.

Heather smiled. She smiled even wider after I carefully reshaped the enamel on two of her overerupted front teeth to bring them back into the line of her smile.

We arranged another visit. I crossed my fingers in true scientific fashion, and waited.

Exactly a month later, Heather returned.

'That tooth you wanted to extract, the one you said you couldn't save, it just fell out,' Heather said.

My heart sank.

'Let's have a look at the rest of your teeth, then,' I said.

Gently, systematically, I used the special periodontal probe to measure the depth of the cuff of gum around each of Heather's teeth.

I shook my head.

'I don't believe it,' I said.

I checked in key areas again.

'That's amazing,' I said.

'What?' Heather asked.

'With the exception of the premolar that fell out, you have a complete remission of your gum disease,' I said.

'I've been doing everything you said. I haven't had a cigarette since I saw you, and I use my cleaning gadgets every day,' Heather said.

'It's working,' I said. 'Now all we need to do is keep you in remission.'

Delighted, I arranged a Smile Whitening Kit to lighten Heather's teeth and a referral to our implant specialist to replace her lost premolar. We gave her smile another even finer cleaning, and updated her oral hygiene gadgets to suit her newly healed gums.

Just a week later, Heather contacted Gentle Dental again.

'Can't thank you enough for everything - not least your Jedi Mind Melt - or whatever you did that convinced me to quit smoking after 40 years!
You are as kind as you are beautiful and my teeth literally could not be in better condition than they are after your treatment.
Look forward to seeing you in June!
Whoever says that to their Dentist?
You are a special person.'

NICOTINE BUSTER

Gianni, an Italian born car salesman, did not pause for breath.

'You've got to clean my teeth. I don't smile anymore. I hate the dentist. I can't work like this. It's been hell...'

Gianni's teeth were covered in dark brown stains. His tongue and the overgrown taste buds on the back third of it where stained brown.

'What part of coffee and cigarettes am I not understanding?' I asked.

'I love them both. I can't start my day without them. Don't ask me to give them up. I need them to keep me sane in my job...' Gianni said.

'The coffee is a cosmetic issue, but the smoking is giving you serious gum disease. You could lose your teeth from smoking, even with impeccable oral hygiene and professional cleaning,' I said.

'But I love my fags. You don't know what it's like in my house first thing in the morning. I have two young children. I adore them, but they're so active...'

'But your smoking doesn't love you back. If you love your children and want to improve your chances of seeing them grow up and have grandchildren, maybe you could consider giving up,' I said, trying a gentle bit of emotional blackmail.

'I'll think about it,' Gianni said, suddenly quiet.

It is my professional duty to make clients aware of the consequences of their habits where their teeth are concerned. It is also my policy to avoid judging, criticizing, shaming, harassing or nagging people. I walk a thin line between speaking up and causing offence, or saying nothing and failing to act in my clients' best interests in preventive health terms.

I dropped the subject while I cleaned Gianni's teeth and affirmed his courage and stamina while we removed the stains and deposits of many years gone by.

Over the next few visits, Gianni had his old black amalgam fillings replaced with white ones. He began to use a tongue scraper. He attended a consultation with the oral surgeon and had his infected wisdom teeth out.

He spoke to anyone and everyone about his dental work. And he sought specialist advice and assistance.

At his first follow up Smile Care Visit, he rolled up his sleeve to show me his new accessory, a nicotine replacement patch.

'My goodness! What happened? Are the kids still alive?' I asked.

'I had to give up. I couldn't undo all your good work, my teeth look so good now, and everything you said made sense,' Gianni said.

'Fantastic. Nicotine replacement therapy doubles your chances of success,' I said.

'Well, I can't go back to smoking now,' Gianni said.

'Oh, that's great,' I said.

'You don't get it,' Gianni said.

'What? Why not?' I asked.

'The guy I see in the pharmacy for the patches, he's not like you. He's scary. He's very tall and he's got big muscles. He said he'd kill me if I go back on the fags. I believe him. I can't say 'no' to him,' Gianni said.

So much for my 'softly, softly' approach. Gianni never smoked again, and continued to do brilliantly at his regular Smile Care Visits.

DRINKING IN MODERATION

Alcohol causes mouth cancer, more so if it is combined with tobacco. The acid in alcohol (like the acid in fizzy drinks) also causes erosion which dissolves the enamel on our teeth. We all know that our teeth, livers and lives improve if we stick to healthy limits when it comes to alcohol. As Alec's story demonstrates, it may also improve the lives of people we socialize with if we stay sober and sensible.

GREAT MATES

'He thought I was looking at his girlfriend the wrong way, so he head butted me,' Alec said.

'Were you?' I asked.

'He was drunk,' Alec said.

'How is he now?' I asked.

'Sober,' Alec said, ' And he's agreed to pay for the damages.'

I took Alec through to the care room, and we examined the cracked tooth in the front of his upper jaw. The injury occurred a week ago on a night out at the pub. Now Alec's central incisor did not respond to cold. It was tender when I tapped it. It had changed to a grey green colour. Over half the crown had disappeared, leaving a diagonal, jagged edge.

'The tooth has died, I'm afraid,' I said.

'I don't want to lose it,' Alec said.

'If we try to save it, it will need a root filling, a post-core, and a crown,' I said.

Alec and I discussed all the alternatives, from doing nothing (free, but disfiguring, unhealthy and uncomfortable), to taking the tooth out and replacing it with an implant (expensive, intrusive and only as a last resort).

'This will be the most expensive pint of beer my mate ever drank,' Alec said as he scheduled his first appointment to begin restoring his tooth.

'Better than having you press charges for assault,' I commented.

'I think that's why he's so happy to pay for the work,' Alec said.

At his next appointment, Alec arrived with his friend.

'Joe's come with me today to pay for my treatment,' he said.

Joe produced a credit card and settled the account.

I sensed tension between Joe and Alec, a mountain of unexpressed feeling between them, perhaps?

'How are you feeling, Joe?' I asked.

'Pretty stupid and sorry,' Joe said.

'Promise me you won't make a habit of this. It's harmful, distressing, and costly,' I said.

'I know. I don't normally,' Joe said. 'I'd just had a bit too much to drink, that's all. When I drink I'm not the same person.'

'He's a great mate, really,' Alec said.

'Ah. Might be a good time to reconsider the value of a wild night out. But if you find you need help to drink less, there are plenty of lovely folk out there to help you. I'll get you some numbers,' I said.

Alec looked approving. Joe looked contrite. I handed Joe the telephone numbers of agencies more experienced in these matters than myself.

After several visits, Alec's tooth was beautifully restored. With the help of my dental laboratory, who examined Alec in person to confirm the shade selection and improve the detailing on his crown, Alec now had a tooth that matched the rest of his smile perfectly.

'Invisible mending,' he said, smiling at himself in the mirror for the first time since his injury had occurred.

I rang Alec some time later to see how he was getting on.

'I don't see Joe that often these days, to tell the truth,' he said.

'Oh,' I said, 'And what about you? How are you and your tooth doing?'

'My new tooth is about to become a celebrity. My band is headlining this summer at that music festival I told you about,' Alec said.

'Well done,' I said, laughing. 'I shall look out for you and your tooth in the line-up.'

DRUGS

Sadly, it's not just cigarettes and alcohol that cause dental damage. As Hitesh's cautionary tale highlights, unless you take your drugs only on your doctor's prescription, they may cause more harm than good.

IT'S NOT CRICKET

The ball flew out of the wicket keeper's hands and up into his face. At over 100km/hr Hitesh didn't stand a chance without a gum shield. And who wears a mouth guard for social cricket? It's not exactly a contact sport.

Hitesh cried out. His hands flew to his mouth. When he removed them a second later, they were covered in blood.

I ran to the stumps from my position in outfield. I like joining in social games, but my lack of any natural sporting ability keeps me on the fringes of most team games. I don't like to let my more competitive teammates down, and in cricket the hardness and speed of the ball scares me.

I looked at Hitesh, with a space where his lower tooth should have been, and felt justified in my fear.

'You're doing great Hitesh,' I said, with what I hoped was reassuring optimism. 'We're going to find your tooth and put it back in.'

Hitesh stayed upright.

My friends and I, moments before either batting or fielding, put down our rivalry and formed a search party for the missing incisor.

'Found it!' said one friend.

'Don't touch it,' I warned. 'It needs handling with care.'

I borrowed a friend's (clean) handkerchief to pick up the tooth by its crown from its nest in the grass.

'Suck this clean,' I instructed Hitesh, who was holding up well.

'Hold open,' I said, gently wriggling the tooth back in its socket.

Hitesh bravely waited with his mouth open while I replanted his tooth.

'Well done,' I said.

'Can we get back to play now?' Hitesh asked.

I hated to disillusion him.

'I'm sorry, Hitesh. We really should go to the hospital and have you checked out.'

'I feel fine now, and we're two wickets down.'

It took a bit of persuading, but eventually, Hitesh, myself, and several of his teammates arrived in the accident and emergency department of the local hospital.

We didn't wait long before being seen, maybe because Hitesh had blood all over his cricket whites.

The oral surgeon on call took us all into a cubicle. An x-ray of Hitesh's jaw was mounted on a viewing screen.

I could see the problem immediately, without a word being said.

A hairline fracture ran through his jaw from the depth of the socket holding his replanted tooth to its lower edge. Hitesh's teeth were covered in calculus, with over half the bone lost in the area of the fracture. His jaw, weakened from gum disease had shattered in the area of impact.

'You've broken your jaw, Hitesh,' I said.

'It's unlikely you'll keep the tooth even though it's been put back so well,' the oral surgeon added.

'When can I play cricket again?' asked Hitesh.

'You'll need antibiotics, soft diet, painkillers and a tetanus booster vaccination,' the oral surgeon replied.

'I feel fine,' Hitesh said.

'And your friend,' the oral surgeon nodded in my direction,' will have to splint your tooth to its neighbours.'

I thanked the oral surgeon as Hitesh and our friends filtered out of the hospital.

Later, I cleaned Hitesh's teeth and fixed his incisors together with resin.

The tooth did not survive. His broken jaw could not sustain the reimplanted incisor without infection, and the tooth was removed again to allow his jaw to heal.

I came to realise that Hitesh was a heavy user of the popular Asian areca products, paan, sopari, tulsi, guthka; he loved to chew them both with and without tobacco. It almost certainly explained his severe gum disease, a complication of regular use in association with poor oral hygiene. I tried to impress upon him the more serious dangers of areca use – mouth scarring and cancer, but to no avail.

I saw Hitesh around a couple more times after his dental trauma, usually when he was standing behind the wicket and it was my reluctant turn to bat.
He never did get his tooth replaced, stop chewing areca or come back for regular dental care.

But he was only 33 years old, in love with his drug of choice and passionate about his cricket.

By now, you may feel you have more than enough items on your self care checklist to keep you occupied for life, but if you want to add road safety and first aid training to your personal health upgrade list, or anything else you know would be helpful all round, why not? If you want further support to improve your lifestyle, consider the NHS Choices website for additional information, and your GP for a general MOT or for attention to any specific health concerns you may have. If you begin all this before your first dental visit, be proud. If not, consider yourself perfectly imperfect, a work of art continually improving and developing over a lifetime. Small steps add up to big changes over time and it's never too late to begin.

MENTAL WELLBEING

Good news! The things that are good for our general wellbeing are also good for our mental wellbeing. Being active and maintaining healthy eating, drinking and sleeping habits is good for both our minds and our bodies. To get our minds into even better condition for our lives and our much awaited dental care, there a few more things we can do to pave the way for our future smiling happiness.

Do Something Fun
Think about what you love doing, lose yourself in, loved doing in the past, or would like to learn. Having fun beats stress, improves our spirits and creates joy, satisfaction and happiness in our lives. Learning new skills gives us a sense of achievement and self-esteem. It would seem obvious, but fun is fun. It is essential for our mental health - and to build our confidence for our exciting dental visits. Go on. Have some fun.

Share, Care and Keep in Touch
Sharing our feelings helps us stay in good mental health and deal with times when we feel troubled. It is good to talk! Caring for others is an important part of staying connected and brings us closer together in our relationships. Keeping in touch with good friends and loving family makes us feel included and cared for. They offer us different views from whatever's going on inside our own heads, keep us active and grounded and help us solve practical problems. In terms of our smile adventures, well-chosen and carefully cultivated family and friends are invaluable.

Distract, Meditate and Relax
A change of scene or a change of pace is good for our mental health. It could be a five-minute pause from cleaning our kitchens, a half-hour lunch break at work or a weekend exploring somewhere new. Even a few minutes of delightful distraction can be enough to de-stress and recharge us for hours.

Meditation and mindfulness involve taking notice and being more aware of the present moment, including our thoughts, bodies and the world around us. It can positively change the way we feel about the world around us and how we approach challenges – including our dental visits.

Relaxation, a wonderful technique to use on our dental visits, is easily learnt, practiced and portable. For more about this, why not try your hand at hypnosis, and just relax...

HYPNOSIS

Hypnosis is a talking treatment that puts you in a relaxed state where you are fully aware and in control of yourself and your physical and mental comfort.

Hypnosis works if you work it, even after a lifetime of dental phobia, and even if you're not sure about it to begin with. Some say it works best if you're intelligent and imaginative – most of us with anxiety are - we're already imagining the worst that can happen, giving ourselves negative suggestions! You just need to be willing and able to 'work it'. Some dentists, like myself, train and practice hypnosis as part of their work. If your chosen dentist does not, a hypnotherapist may help. Many qualified hypnotherapists work with people with dental anxiety and phobias and are able to help you prepare for fear free dental visits. Or, you could 'do it yourself'...

Feel free to practice the following self-hypnosis technique at home until it becomes second nature. You can even record the words below in your best 'bedtime story voice' and play them back to yourself as you prepare for your dental visits. During your self hypnosis, holding your thumb and forefinger together creates a physical 'anchor' and your positive phrase becomes an affirmation to use to relax and support your mind and body during your actual dental visit. It's as easy as lying back and imagining...

SELF HYPNOSIS

Make yourself comfortable, as comfortable as you can.

Now relax the muscles around your eyes, to the point where those eye muscles won't work and your eyes gently close and stay closed. And when you're sure your eye muscles won't work, test them and make sure they won't work. That's great. Now let that feeling you have in your eye muscles go all the way down to your toes. Cover yourself with a blanket of relaxation.

Notice how good you feel just because you've got this amount of relaxation. And every time you open and close your eyes your relaxation doubles. So now, open your eyes, and close them again. Let yourself completely relax. This is excellent physical relaxation.

Now we're going to relax your mind to the point where you are just as relaxed mentally as you are physically.

In a moment you will start counting backwards from one hundred, and with each number you say aloud, you'll double the relaxation you had at the previous number. By the time you get through a few numbers you'll be so relaxed mentally you won't be able to think of numbers, the numbers just won't be there.

Now start counting, out loud. Double your relaxation with each number, and just watch the numbers disappear. Just watch them go. Watch them disappear completely... Going, gone completely, aren't they?

That's great. Notice how good you feel when this mental and physical relaxation together takes hold. Just let it take hold. With every breath you take now, that relaxation is going to become more intense.

Now imagine you're at the dentist and by some miracle your anxiety has disappeared.

You feel great. You walk in confidently. Your dentist is your friend. You feel safe and loved and cared for. You are in command of your breathing, speaking and swallowing.

You sit comfortably in the dental chair. You are surrounded by love and care and trusted expertise. You are in the driver's seat, assertive and in control. Your dentist listens to you and follows your instructions safely and surely.

Nothing disturbs you. Nothing distracts you. You know that all the sensations you feel are part of your successful dental care. Nothing disturbs or distracts you. You sit back and enjoy the experience while your smile is beautifully and comfortably restored to dazzling perfection.

Now you are holding on to this good feeling, this safe and happy feeling of relaxation and love and safety.

And while you are holding onto this great feeling, I want you to touch your left thumb and forefinger together and keep a simple phrase of your own choosing in mind, to remind yourself of this great experience and to bring it back for you at any time in the future.

Keep your left thumb and forefinger touching and gently say this phrase out loud...

That's great! Any time in future you touch your left thumb and forefinger together, you will be able to feel this wonderful feeling of relaxation and love and confidence and safety, at any time or place you need.
In a moment, you're going to count to five to bring yourself out of hypnosis. When you do this you will feel increasingly awake and your eyes will reopen. You will remember everything you have heard and said and you will feel relaxed and refreshed.

One... slowly, calmly, easily, gently, you are returning to full awareness again.

Two... each muscle and nerve in your body is loose and relaxed and you feel wonderfully relaxed.

Three... from head to toe you feel good in every way, physically, mentally and emotionally, calm and serene.

Four... your eyes begin to feel sparkling clear.

Five... your eyelids open, you are fully aware, awake, calm, rested, refreshed relaxed, invigorated and full of energy.

Open your eyes. Take a deep breath, fill up your lungs and stretch.

Well done. You've done brilliantly. You'll always be able to take that relaxation with you, for all your dental visits.

Ask for Help

We all sometimes get tired or overwhelmed by how we feel or when things go wrong. If we're not sure if things are getting too much for us, asking our loved ones how we seem or checking online for quick and easy mental health screening questionnaires for anxiety and/or depression, for example, can tell us if it's time to seek professional help.

Accept Ourselves

Some of us make people laugh, some of us are good at maths and some of us cook fantastic meals. We are all different. As is the case for Frank in our next story, acceptance is the key to embracing our unique qualities and appreciating the wonder of each and every one of us.

PYRAMID SELLING

I first met Frank when he came with his mother to a dental appointment. His teeth needed a good clean, but were otherwise in excellent condition.

'What do you do when you're not here at the dentist?' I asked.

'I do a lot of graphic design and computer work,' Frank said.

'Who do you work for?' I asked.

'No-one. I'm on disability benefit,' Frank said.

'Oh,' I said. 'What's wrong with you?'

'I have mental health problems,' Frank said.

'What kind?' I asked. I have a keen interest in mental health, from both the consumer and provider angles.

'My psychiatrist says it's a bit like schizophrenia, what I have,' Frank said.

'Okay. Well, if you're ever not feeling well, let me know so we can help,' I said.

I'm accustomed to making the occasional call to psychiatric health care workers to coordinate care and appointments. I tell anorexic clients to eat because I don't want them to die after all the beautiful dental work we've done. I tell clients with suicidal thoughts to ring me if they feel like killing themselves, and I'll say, 'no'. I discuss how antidepressants and talking treatments keep me (relatively) sane and happy, and in doing so stay real, connected and useful.

Once, a client with schizophrenia invited his ward mate to my practice. The friend, in the unfamiliar environment, suffered a paranoid outburst. I offered him a glass of water while we then waited, with calm and dignity, for the police. No one was hurt or offended. He was readmitted for inpatient care. He had stopped taking his tablets because of the side effects, it later transpired. He returned looking much better when he was stabilized with a new medication.

Frank, however, was never ill enough to require medication, nor well enough to work in paid employment. He lived a nocturnal life, working on his computer by night and sleeping by day.

After some years, I became familiar with Frank's routine and his interesting worldview. He took to wearing a metal pyramid on his head and an amulet around his neck.

'What are they for?' I asked.

'They keep the evil spirits away,' Frank said.

'Really? Where did you get them?' I asked.

'You have to get them off the internet. They're not widely available,' Frank said.

'How much did you pay for them?' I asked.

'Four hundred pounds,' Frank said.

'Wow,' I said. 'How long do they last?'

'Well, I've had the amulet forever,' Frank said, showing us the golden nugget with its ruby stone on the gold chain around his neck. 'I don't take it off.'

Indeed, it looked very solid.

'But I do need a new pyramid,' Frank said. 'This one is wearing out at the soldered joints, and it won't work if it's broken.'

'Please do be careful to get your money's worth,' I said. 'You want something stronger if you get a replacement.'

I do feel concerned at the vulnerability of people with mental illness. Was I wrong not to dissuade Frank from the purchase of any kind of talisman? I'm still not sure. Like horseshoes, rabbit's feet and four leaf clovers, Frank's pyramid brought him a sense of security. Who am I to judge another person's paradigm, let alone their pyramid?

In the process of improving our mental health, there is one more important step we may take to get our heads in order – healing any shame that adds to our understandable dental dillying, dallying and delaying.

Healing Shame

Alongside our dental fears often comes shame, and fear of shame. Shame is the felt belief that we are somehow bad. We all have 'good' and 'bad' parts of ourselves, our thoughts and our feelings. For the sake of convenience and the common good, however, our conscientious parents and polite society may attempt to keep us on our best 'good' behaviour with words that are unfortunately shaming.

Before around four years of age, children are considered 'precooperative' in developmental and behavioural terms. Not 'uncooperative', but 'precooperative'; not unwilling, but unable, to comply with instructions. Trying to force tiny children to overcome their natural reflexes or instincts is a losing battle, as any parent of a toddler will tell you. If we, as tiny children, are belittled, shouted at, or threatened with dire consequences for not doing as a caregiver (or should I say 'scaregiver') instructs, we may develop fear and shame.

If, as children, we are told to 'be good at the dentist', and we aren't, if we are compared to other 'well-behaved' children and found lacking, we may develop shame. If as children, we suffer dental pain or inadequate dental care, and simply felt it must be 'our fault' rather than acknowledging the scary truth that sometimes our caregivers are imperfect or even negligent or cruel, we may develop shame.

If as children and adults, we are told to 'stop coughing, stay still, lie down, or, be quiet' at the dentist, we may develop shame. If, when we finally pluck up the courage to visit a dentist, we are told, 'you should have come sooner', or, 'your teeth are in a terrible state', we may develop shame. If we put off going to the dentist while our teeth and gums slide further and further into difficulty, our shame may increase to the point where we develop a shame phobia, making it even harder to seek care for fear of 'being told off'. If, when we try to explain our fears and reactions, we are told, 'you shouldn't think/feel/say/do that', no matter how well meaning, we may develop or increase our shame.

But our mouths connect us to food, water and air, our primary sources of life. Dentists poke around in our mouths, the unconscious seat of our first infant experiences of survival – and love. Our reflexes, coughing, gagging, moving and making noise, are normal and healthy reactions, designed to protect our airways and our feeding tubes.

Our dental fears and phobias may be constitutional or learned and have origins in our biological drive for survival. Our 'cowardice' is actually a deep-seated desire for life. It does rather make the idea of having dental phobias seem, well, logical, doesn't it?

Despite all the very good reasons for dental fears and phobias, sometimes our shame is so entrenched that we continue the process of unwittingly shaming ourselves, like Mary, below.

SHAME

'My teeth are in an awful state,' Mary said.

'Let's have a look together,' I said, passing Mary the hand mirror.

'I don't want to look,' Mary said.

We looked together.

'We'll give your teeth a really good spring clean. Otherwise, they're doing really well,' I said.

'I should have come sooner,' Mary said.

'You're here now,' I said. 'That's great.'

I cleaned Mary's teeth to sparkling perfection and invited her to inspect them while I demonstrated the finer points of flossing. Mary looked at her teeth critically.

'I'm sorry I let them get like this,' Mary insisted.

'Actually, they're not too bad,' I said.

'I know it's my fault. I should have looked after them better,' Mary said.

'Well, you do have lots of fillings, but your teeth seem very stable now,' I said.

'I must be your worst patient,' Mary said.

'My worst patients are the ones who never make it through the door,' I assured her. 'You've shown a lot of courage coming here today.'

'I don't know about that,' Mary said.

Mary, a 54 -year-old university administrator, was suffering from chronic dental shame.

'How long have you blamed yourself for the condition of your teeth?' I asked.

Mary looked at me, surprised.

'I'm sure you didn't want or cause all your fillings, and yet you hold yourself completely responsible for them,' I said.

'I know they're my fault. I should have eaten less sweets,' Mary said.

'Some people eat loads of sweets, and they never get any holes in their teeth. Other people get decay because of the bacteria in their mouths or because their tooth enamel is weaker, ' I said.

'But it's all preventable,' Mary protested.

'Sure, but I bet you didn't know that when you were young. Most children eat the sweets their parents or grandparents buy them, and it's a hard habit to give up,' I said.

'My Mum ate sweets, too. She lost all her teeth in her forties,' Mary remembered.

'At least you've got teeth to complain about,' I said, 'so you're doing better than your Mum.'

'And my children are doing better than me. I gave them less sweets. I took them to the dentist regularly when they were young and they've hardly got any fillings.'

'You do care about your teeth, and your children's. When did you say your last visit to the dentist was?' I asked.

'Four years ago. I was frightened of being told off. I was looking around for a dentist that seemed kind and the time just got longer and longer. Then I saw your website.'

'Well, you've done brilliantly today. Thank you for putting your trust in us.'

Mary and I talked about cosmetic options for her heavily restored teeth; white fillings, veneers, smile whitening and crown and bridgework. We discussed using affirmations to heal her shame, and her fear of shame, around her teeth.

Mary made an appointment to begin her cosmetic work.

Later in the day, I visited my hairdresser. Despite my general fear of hairdressers, I liked this lady, a kind, talented young stylist who was also working to put herself through business school.

I sat down in her swivel chair.

'My hair is in an awful state. I should have come sooner,' I said.

If we were shamed for our fears and protective behaviours in the past, chances are we now continue the job ourselves, telling ourselves how to 'behave' and giving ourselves a 'telling off' with sentences containing the shame laden 'should' word.

'I should drink more water.'

'I shouldn't drink so much.'

'I should stop smoking.'

'I should eat less sweets.'

'I should floss my teeth.'

'I shouldn't have left it so long.'

'I shouldn't be such a coward.'

'I should be much better at the dentist.'

'I should get my teeth fixed.'

Etc. etc. etc.

PLEASE STOP.

Shaming language is the enemy of self-esteem, growth and change. Even ordinary guilt or regret (which encourages us to improve our actions) is preferable to the shame that leads us feel bad about ourselves and increases the risk that we will avoid the very situations we need to confront and change. But it is possible to 'mind our language' and reframe negative shaming thoughts with positive affirming words.

So humour me. Just for fun, take the above prescriptions, and turn them into affirmations, simply by swapping the 'should' word for something kinder.

'I'd like to drink more water.'

'I'm ready to cut down on my drinking.'

'I'd love to stop smoking.'

'I'd like to eat more healthily.'

'I'd like to floss my teeth.'

'I'd prefer not to have left it so long.'

'I'm my favourite coward.'

'I'd like to be much better at the dentist.'

'I would love to get my teeth fixed.'

And so on. Feel free to add in your own examples, keeping them as real, open, honest and true for yourself as possible. Read your affirmations aloud, pin them up with post-it notes and share them with your supporters.

How does that feel? Affirmations transform paralyzing shame into the loving intentions we need to help us on our journey. While we're using fear-busting and non-shaming words and language to positively shape our thoughts and feelings, why don't we consider making the following substitutions to improve our confidence even further.

Oldspeak (scary/shaming) (friendly/shame free)	**Newspeak**
Dental appointment	Dental visit
The dentist	My dentist
Waiting room	Lounge room
Dental chair chair	Driver's seat/ Magic

Behave/ be good signals	Speak / Use stop
Horrible sore/ugly wound	Impressive lesion
Bad teeth	VIP teeth
Bad gums	VIP gums
Bad breath challenge	Fresh breath
Decay/ cavities/ holes	Filling opportunities
Open wide together	Let's have a little look
Bad gagging	Good gag reflex
Small mouth formed mouth	Small and perfectly
Big mouth	Beautiful access
Scaler polishing wand	Magic cleaning and
Topical anaesthetic	Magic jelly
Injection/ Needle	Magic sleepy juice
Drill	Magic cleaning wand
Rubber dam	Tooth blanket
White Filling	Invisible mending
Pain	Discomfort

Stop break	Have a commercial
Extract the tooth	Deliver the tooth

Words are powerful things. We can use them to express our thoughts and values – and they can shape our thoughts and values too. We can use our creative language power for good. Whenever a new word or phrase feels more supportive and safe, feel free to use it. This is not to silence our fears with inappropriate euphemisms, but to give us a way to calm our agitated inner children when we are contemplating our dental care. Having now worked to accept our feelings and to avoid shaming ourselves, we continue our quest to seek out affirming experiences, and if this fails, to follow the example of Sandra below, and refuse to accept inappropriate shame if it is offered to us.

PAIN IN THE NECK

Sandra, a statuesque ash blonde in her sixties, had a lot of responsibility in her life. She managed and cared for many people in an elder care home. She looked after her feisty but largely dependent mother. She trained as a spiritual healer in her 'spare' time.

Now she was here, finally, to look after herself.

'How did you find us?' I asked her.

'I went to a dentist who said I was an, 'awful nuisance', because I have a bad neck and couldn't get comfortable in the dental chair,' Sandra said.

'What did you do?' I asked.

'I said, 'Not for much longer', got out of his dental chair and left,' Sandra said.

Sandra explained she later met a dental student who affirmed her for having special needs, and suggested she find a dentist with interest and experience in meeting such challenges. She researched online and found my website.

Over many visits, I learned that Sandra's mother was highly demanding and had refused nursing home care, which was why her loving but often exasperated daughter now looked after her. Indeed, her work at the care home felt easier than caring for her mother. I tried to be supportive.

It did not surprise me when Sandra asked not to be lain too far back in the dental chair because of her neck problems. I wondered if her 'pain in the neck' was a physical expression of the feelings she might have about carrying so much 'weight on her shoulders'.

I spent some time restoring Sandra's broken and missing teeth and giving her back confidence in her smile. Whenever I laid the dental chair back, we would always stop early or adjust the position and headrest for her comfort. Sandra was instructed to raise her hand during treatment if she needed anything, including a break just to move about and prevent her neck from stiffening up.

When Sandra revealed at a subsequent visit that the pain in her neck was much improved, I could not help wondering if she had retired from the care home, finished her training, or even, God forgive me, if her mother had died. I marvelled at Sandra's newfound ease with the fully reclined position of the dental chair.

'What has changed in your life to bring about this miracle?' I asked, sharing my thoughts with Sandra.

Sandra assured me she was still working, training, and engaging with her very much alive mother. Far from having a psychological cause, Sandra's neck problems were the legacy of four separate motorbike and car crash whiplash injuries involving joy riders, police, an ex-husband and bad luck.

'I've found a marvellous chiropractor,' she said. 'He spent some time adjusting my neck and it's made a huge difference.'

I congratulated Sandra on her transformation – and, just in case I needed it in the future, asked her for the name of her chiropractor.

Well, then. We've shored up our general and mental health and are ready for more… hopefully. If not, keep working the previous steps until you feel more prepared. If you are ready, it's time to get your teeth into the next step of our self-care strategy.

DENTAL WELLBEING

Imagine you hire a cleaner. Do you invite them in, declare that you don't know where the cleaning equipment is, ignore all the stuff on your floor and sit down with a cup of tea while your newest domestic team member tries to put your house in order? Okay, okay, maybe that's just me… And that's fine, but I do understand that tidying up before a cleaner arrives and making sure the cleaning cupboard is well stocked is a time honoured tradition for a reason. It is designed to maintain our homes between professional cleans, to allow our cleaners to focus on the heavy stuff that we find harder to get around to, and probably, let's be honest, to reduce our domestic shame sufficiently so that we're willing to let a complete stranger into our homes. Putting our preventive dental programs into action before our dental visits does the same thing for our mouths. It reduces our shame, improves our oral health, and clears the way for our dentists to tackle the tough stuff.

Need more motivation? In an ideal world, we would all want to keep our teeth sparkling clean for health reasons. In the real world, most of us, like Rodney, below, simply want to look our best and feel attractive. And when vanity and cosmetic care can safely boost our appearance, self-esteem and health, that's got to be good.

WHITER THAN WHITE

'How much do you charge for tooth whitening?' the young man asked.

He had walked in off the street to make the enquiry.

I named our fee, reading from the fee scale posted at the reception counter.

The man looked excited.

'Is it for yourself?' I asked.

'Yes,' he said.

'I'm sorry,' I said. 'I can't do it for you.'

'Why not?' I heard the protest in his voice.

'Your teeth are already very white. You don't need them whitened.'

'But I do,' he said.

'Look,' I said, 'I'd be the first to tell you if they needed lightening. I love our Smile Whitening Kit. It's the safest and most effective method available. And I'd hate to miss a commercial opportunity. But your teeth are really very white already,' I said.

'You won't make me one of your Smile Whitening Kit thingys?' he asked.

'No,' I said.

'But my ex-girlfriend said my teeth were yellow,' he said, leaning forward, opening his mouth, showing me his teeth.

'Ah,' I said.

'Just before she dumped me by text,' he said.

'Ah,' I said. 'I think I can explain.'

I whipped out our shade guide from the cupboard and invited the young man to look in the mirror on top of the reception counter.

'This is your shade,' I said, holding up a tab next to his upper central incisor for comparison.

He nodded in agreement.

I took the tab and placed it back in the shade guide.

'Can you see that your shade is lighter than A1, the lightest shade we have?' I asked.

'Yeah,' the man said. 'So it is.'

He paused.

'What was she on about, then?' he asked.

'I'm Kathy, the dentist, by the way,' I said, avoiding the question.

'Rodney, my name's Rodney,' the young man said.

We shook hands.

'Rodney,' I said, 'Your teeth don't need whitening, but they do need cleaning.'

'What's the difference?' Rodney asked.

'Whitening changes the colour of the tooth itself – which you don't need,' I said.

Rodney nodded.

'Cleaning gets rid of built up plaque, calculus and surface stains,' I said.

'And that's what I need?' Rodney asked.

Ah, the tricky bit.

'Definitely. The reason you have bad breath is because your teeth need cleaning. And we need to get you cleaning at home, with floss, probably,' I said.

'You're saying I have bad breath?' Rodney asked.

'Well, yes. I only notice it when you lean right in,' I said, trying to be tactful.

'How come no one ever told me?' Rodney asked.

'Well, it's my job to notice these things and tell people,' I said. 'To be honest, most people know someone with bad breath, but very few people actually tell them.'

'You know what? I think my ex-girlfriend was trying to,' Rodney said. 'I wish she'd told me sooner.'

'Would it have made a difference?' I asked.

'It might have,' Rodney said. 'But if it didn't, at least I would have got my teeth cleaned, and then plenty of women would be interested in me, I bet.'

'It's never too late. Let's book you in and get you all spring cleaned, and then you can find out,' I said.

Don't worry if you're confused by all the dental health gadgets they sell in your local pharmacy or which electric toothbrush to buy. As a professional I'm not allowed to recommend any specific brand of oral health product, but as an individual with sensitive teeth and challenging gums, I can share that I prefer a simple rechargeable electric toothbrush with a rotating head (soft, of course), high fluoride toothpaste, broad, soft dental floss/tape (I have been known to use white plumbers' tape, PTFE, for this with great success) and interdental brushes to meet my daily high maintenance oral hygiene requirements. I choose a U-shaped metal scraper for cleaning my tongue, I brush the roof of my mouth, and I rinse with a 0.2% chlorhexidine gluconate mouthrinse for one minute by the clock if my gums flare up.

If you have bridgework or orthodontic wires, I can also recommend a unique nylon monofilament, aka, 'fishing line', for threading under bridges and archwires and gaining access to floss tricky interdental areas. Yes, really. Yet another example of my best lateral thinking moments, if I do say so myself. If you wear dentures, removable orthodontic appliances, a sports guard/gumshield, night guard or mouth splint, please make a habit of soaking in a specialist denture care solution, brushing and rinsing your kit after use. Do not keep dentures (false teeth) in your lovely mouth all day and night – our mouths need a rest to stay healthy.

And another thing... Tongue jewellery... Oral piercings can lead to life threatening infections. Inhaled separated fragments may require chest surgery to remove. Not attractive. Make your Mum and Dad happy and don't get one, or remove any you do have. And if your Mum or Dad are the ones with oral piercings, ask them to remove them. Tell them I said so.

Our gums may bleed a little, or even a lot, the first few times we offer them all this unaccustomed care. Don't be put off by this. Use plaque disclosing tablets or solutions to identify any areas that need more attention. As this bleeding reduces, it is a sure sign that our gums are grateful for our newfound diligence and plaque removal. Keep it up. This daily debridement adds up to a lifetime of fresh breath and helps us keep most, if not all, of our teeth, forever.

23 TEETH

When I first met Mrs James, she was in her sixties. I was in my early thirties. I greeted her by her first name.

'I prefer to be called, "Mrs James",' she advised me.

Chastened, I obliged.

Over time, and countless regular visits, I got to know Mrs James a little. She seemed reserved by my relaxed hybrid English-Australian-global standards. We chatted about children after mine was born, and she shared briefly about her two daughters. I mentioned my divorce and introduced her to my new partner. She always visited with her husband, Mr James, a war veteran and her lifelong partner. They were inseparable and obviously in love.

Nothing stays the same, it is said.

The first time I saw Mrs James cry, briefly, was when she took me aside after one appointment to explain that Mr James had developed dementia, and was increasingly forgetful. The man she loved was disappearing, replaced by another with round the clock dependency needs.

Mr and Mrs James continued their regular visits, until the day Mrs James came alone. The second time I saw Mrs James cry was when she told me Mr James had passed away.

Every six months, without fail, Mrs James attended the practice for her routine Smile Care Visit. Check up, clean and fluoride. Mrs James, and her teeth, were among the strongest and most stable influences in my life. If I had any questions about life, the universe or anything, from recipes to romance, I could ask Mrs James.

When Mrs James' eldest daughter became ill with terminal cancer, Mrs James did miss a dental appointment – to visit her daughter and her family one more time. At the next appointment, remembering her daughter's life and passing, we both shared the tissue box.

By now, Mrs James had indicated that it would be fine for me to call her by her first name. When I occasionally did, it felt uncomfortable, its informality somehow lacking in the respect I felt she deserved.

Three years ago, Mrs James arrived for her visit with severe bruising of her face and limbs. She had taken a tumble whilst running for a bus.

'I am eighty one, I do not run,' her younger daughter had exhorted her to say to herself if she felt the urge to run in future.

I agreed with her daughter. And after that appointment, whenever it was possible, my partner chauffeured Mrs James home.

Last week, Mrs James arrived with a present of home made Seville orange ('Is there any other kind?' she asked) marmalade.

During her appointment, she invited me to count her teeth.

'Twenty three teeth,' she exclaimed. 'That's one less than my daughter!'

'This preventive dentistry stuff works. You're doing well,' I replied.

'We're doing well,' she said.

When Mrs James left, I held the jar of marmalade, my transitional object, and felt my love for her.

Life may have many losses, but some things, not just teeth and health, do endure and grow.

So. There you have it, the essentials of sensational self-care that will stand us in good stead throughout our dental visits and for the whole of our lifetimes beyond. If you have managed to get this far, well done. If you are still too frightened to make a start, do not be too concerned. A loving dentist will help us with these steps when we see them. It's time now for us to go forth and visit our chosen dentists, keeping in mind, respectfully, our cherished (or not) dental fears and phobias.

Chapter 9.

Lift off!

We have gained support, made a dental appointment and improved our general, mental and dental self-care.

Now we consider how to manage on our actual visits. First, let's take a little look at a visit from a dentist's point of view. Knowledge is power. Knowing more of what to expect from our dentists, with the help of a small glimpse into a dentist's 'practice ritual' (mine in this case), might be very reassuring.

SEE YOU IN SIX MONTHS

If your dentist is anything like me they may have developed a 'script' for welcoming, treating and farewelling their clients with a minimum of fuss and a maximum of cheer on their regular visits. It might go something like this...

'Hello, Mr(s) Smith. How are you?'

'Please take a seat, I'll just be a moment.'

'Would you like to follow me?'

'Make yourself comfortable.'

'Any change to your health since you were last here?'

'How are your teeth and gums behaving?'

'How are you managing with the dental floss?'

'How was your holiday?'

'Let's have a look at you... wow! Your teeth are gorgeous...'

'Your home care is excellent.'

'Upper right eight, seven, six, five...'

'Your teeth are doing brilliantly and your gums and soft tissues are great!'

'All you need is a routine spring clean.'

'Pop your hand up if you need a commercial break... most of my clients prefer breathing to dentistry.'

'Sorry about all the prodding and poking... you're doing great.'

'Just a little polish now.'

'Have a really good rinse.'

'Have a look in the mirror. Your teeth are beautiful. How do they feel?'

'May I give you a fluoride treatment?'

'Nothing to eat, rinse or drink for half an hour, if that's okay.'

'Well done! Your mouth is very stable. 'Stable' sounds so much better than 'boring' don't you think?'

'I'll see you in six months.'

'How would you like to pay?'

'Thank you very much. That's lovely.'

'Here's your receipt. Let's schedule your next appointment.'

'How does 10am on Thursday the 25th of September sound?'

'I'll just write that down for you.'

'How do you think Spurs will do in the Premier League this season?'

'No, me neither, but I live in hope.'

'Lovely to see you again. Take care. See you soon.'

There. Easy. (If you're a dentist, or dental student reading this, by the way, feel free to vary the script according to your own personality, circumstances, and those of your clients.)

If, like me, your dentist has a customary patter, replying in kind will add to your sense of security as this timeless practice ritual is acted out with its very own brand of reassuring continuity.

If, on the other hand, you feel mischievous and in need of a change, try giving the following responses...

'I'm not well, otherwise I wouldn't be here.'

'Why do I have to wait? I'm here on time.'

'No, I wouldn't like to follow you.'

'How can I possibly make myself comfortable in a dental chair?'

'I'm getting older, can't you tell?'

'If my teeth and gums could look after themselves I wouldn't need to be here.'

'You can floss my teeth for me, that's your job.'

'I'll need a holiday after this.'

'Just get on with it.'

'Call yourself 'Gentle Dental'?'

'My teeth look the same as they always do. What do you mean?'

'I hate fluoride. It tastes disgusting.'

'Of course my teeth are stable. I come here every six months, don't I?'

'I wouldn't like to pay.'

'Who said I want to come back?'

'Spurs? I'm an Arsenal supporter.'

'I'd like to say it was lovely seeing you too... but I can't.'

See how much fun you can have at your dental visit? Let me know how you get on. I'll see you in six months.

Name your fear

So, you now have a general understanding of what might typically happen on your regular visits to your dentist – and even how you might add a bit of repartee when you feel like it. On the basis that knowledge is power, it may also help to know how dentists go about planning treatment. Although I can't speak for all my colleagues, in my delightful (yes!) care protocols, stage one is relief of any pain, stage two is control of infection e.g. fillings, root fillings if required and hygiene, stage three is long term restoration e.g. crowns, bridges, implants and cosmetic work, and stage four is preventive maintenance e.g. regular reviews, hygiene and fluoride treatments. Stage three is considered elective, and usually depends on the successful completion of the first two stages. Some of us only go to the dentist for crisis intervention (stage one care) rather than planned maintenance (all stages), which is more likely to keep us in beautiful good health while we enjoy trouble free dental motoring. If this sounds familiar, stay with me. The aim of this book is to help us get ourselves further along the smile care spectrum.

But maybe I'm getting ahead of myself. Most importantly for us dental delayers and dodgers, we need to feel reassured from our very first visits. This is where knowing about ourselves, our special care needs, and the ways we can cope with them is vital. The next step in fixing our phobias is, wherever possible, to 'find' our fears. This provides us with esteem boosting validation and will help our dentists to tailor our care accordingly.

Dentists interested in caring for anxious people like us will ask about our phobias, how and when they started, and what triggers them now. Those of us with a sensitive gag reflex or blocked sinuses may be terrified of choking. Those of us with vertigo may experience extreme dizzy spells if our heads are turned to the side while we are lying down or if the dental chair is put back or up without warning. Others of us have needle phobias, blood phobias, swallowing phobias, or histories of assault, domestic violence or sexual abuse, all of which we need to acknowledge and work with and through.

Identifying and naming your fears will give you the extra affirmation and information you need to move forward in your sensational smile recovery. If the experiences shared in this chapter do not remind you of your own situation, do not despair. If these stories seem more or less extreme than your own, remember it is not necessarily the type or extent of our wounds that determines our wellbeing but how we perceive and respond to them. Each of us has our own unique story. It is the spirit of willingness to overcome our challenges that is important here. As you read further, take what you like, add your own tricks and techniques, and leave the rest. Use whatever works for you. Go for it!

GENERAL FEARS

LOSS OF CONTROL PHOBIA

Many of us fear losing control, whether it is through drink, drugs, illness, being on lifts, escalators, trains or aeroplanes, and on any occasion where we put our well being into the hands of others. At the dentist, this can manifest as a dread of sedation or general anaesthetic (GA). Sometimes, this fear is for a very good reason. Fortunately, there are alternatives to pharmacological management of dental anxiety, as was the case for Andrew.

CHEATING DEATH

'I know my teeth are in pretty bad shape. I should have come years ago.'

'You're here now. That's got to be good,' I said.

'It's too late now. They all need to come out. I was planning early retirement when Robert Maxwell stole my pension. I kept working and never got time to see the dentist,' Andrew explained.

'That's okay. We'll look at you together and make a plan,' I said.

Andrew lay back while I checked his whole mouth carefully.

'Any thoughts on giving up smoking?' I asked.

'None. I love my smoking,' Andrew said.

'Okay. I'm duty bound to advise you on the joys of being smoke free. Let me know if you change your mind,' I smiled.

'Not likely,' Andrew said.

'We will need an x-ray to check the bone levels around your teeth, but it does look as though you are struggling with gum disease,' I said.

Andrew's x-ray of all his teeth and jaws was available on the computer soon after.

'It's not good news, I'm afraid,' I said, shaking my head.

'I thought not,' Andrew nodded.

'There's been a lot of hidden bone loss, smoking related. Most of the teeth only have a few millimetres of bone left holding them in. That's why they've been moving,' I said.

'Okay,' Andrew said.

'I'm sorry,' I said.

'I knew they'd all have to come out,' Andrew said.

'Even if you stopped smoking today, the bone loss has gone so far, you would almost certainly keep losing teeth,' I said.

'I don't want to be in and out of here for the next ten years. I have a business to run,' Andrew said.

'We could take all your remaining teeth out with local anaesthetic. It does take several appointments, and we need to work with our denture technician to get you immediate false teeth,' I said.

'That's great. As long as it's not a general,' Andrew said unexpectedly.

'You said you don't like the dentist on the 'phone when we made your appointment. A lot of people with dental phobias ask for general anaesthetic or sedation. How come you prefer local anaesthetic?' I asked.

'The last time I had a general anaesthetic for an extraction was thirty years ago. I was very ill. I couldn't walk properly for a week afterwards, I was so sick. Then I found out the dentist I saw was later convicted of killing someone with general anaesthetic,' Andrew said.

'Sounds like you were a near miss. That would put me off general anaesthetics and dentists for life,' I said.

'It took a lot to get me through your door, I can tell you,' Andrew said.

'You'll be pleased to know that general anaesthetics in dentistry without qualified anaesthetists were banned in 1992, because of avoidable deaths in general practice,' I said.

'I am very pleased,' Andrew said.

We both agreed to keep it safe and simple. Andrew had all his remaining teeth removed with local anaesthetic in three visits. His immediate dentures fitted well. He looked even better than before treatment.

When I called Andrew two days after his last visit, he was grateful, alive and well, and back at work.

MESS/ INFECTION PHOBIA/ OCD

Sometimes, our fears combine with other phobias or OCD
(Obsessive Compulsive Disorder) and make it harder for us to
receive dental care. Speaking to our doctors about these phobias,
thoughts and behaviours can help us get the treatment we need
to improve our lives generally. If, like Jon, below, you find dental
visits difficult as well, a little bit of extra help from your support
team might make all the difference.

MUM POWER

Jon was only thirty-four years old, exceptionally shy, single, and
struggling. He did not like the dentist, but his teeth were loose
and painful. Reluctantly, he had made an appointment.

'I don't want any teeth out,' he said.

'Let's just have a look, and then we'll talk about it together,' I
said.

I ran a periodontal probe, a depth gauge for gums, gently around
Jon's teeth. The numbers told a bleak story. Jon had a very
aggressive kind of gum disease.

'It's not good news I'm afraid,' I said.

Jon waited.

'Normally there is a gap of two or three millimeters between the
gum and the tooth,' I said. 'But when there is infection, it
deepens, until there's not enough gum or bone left to hold the
tooth in the jaw.'

Jon sat very still.

'At least a quarter of your teeth have lost over a centimeter of attachment to the gum. That's why they're feeling loose and sore.'

Jon spoke for the first time.

'I brush my teeth four times a day,' he said.

'You do a great job of brushing. Maybe too good a job in places, that's why your teeth are sensitive, because some of the enamel is worn away. But you will need to clean between your teeth as well. And see me for professional cleaning every three months.'

'What can you do about the teeth that are loose?' Jon asked.

'I'm sorry, Jon. We can't give you back what you've already lost. Your gum disease is very serious. You may even lose some teeth, but we'll try to save as many as we can for as long as we can,' I said.

'I don't want any teeth out,' Jon repeated.

I referred Jon to a specialist postgraduate dental teaching hospital. They wrote back after a thorough round of assessment and intensive hygiene treatment, nominating six teeth for extraction which were beyond salvation – the same teeth we had identified as severely affected by gum disease on his first visit. They asked me to remove them to improve the chances of Jon's remaining teeth and gums staying healthy and pain free.

Jon refused.

'I don't want extractions,' he said.

This time, I waited. I gave Jon an antibiotic prescription in case any of his periodontal pockets, the deep gaps between his gums and teeth, flared up with infection over a holiday or weekend. I advised him not to hesitate to call if necessary.

The telephone rang one month later.

'I can't stand it any more. My gums hurt too much. I want the extractions,' Jon said.

We made Jon an appointment. Then, on the day of his visit, Jon balked.

'I can't have them out,' he said. 'I'm scared. I need to use the toilet.'

John disappeared into the loo. Ten minutes passed. Concerned, I approached the door. I could hear the sounds of running water from the hand basin. Gently, I knocked on the door.

'John, are you okay?' I asked.

'Yes,' John answered.

The sound of running water stopped. The door opened and John emerged.

'It's my OCD. I have to wash my hands,' John explained.

'That's okay,' I said.

We sat down in the consultation area again. I spent some time selling the benefits of extractions to Jon, reassuring him that the anaesthetic meant he wouldn't feel a thing, praising him for his courage, telling him I knew he could do it, we would be there for him, he would feel better afterwards. I tried everything I could think of.

'I'm too scared. Just give me the antibiotics. I'll have to try again another day,' Jon said.

I reminded Jon that antibiotics were a holding measure only –
that's why he was here now. If he had the teeth out today, he
would be fixed.

'I can't,' Jon said.

Then I remembered Jon's mother. Unmarried, he lived at home
with his widowed mother.

'Let's call your mum,' I said.

I spoke to Jon's mother, explaining the situation, and passed the
'phone to Jon.
After two minutes, Jon got back in the dental chair.

'I'm ready now,' he said.

The anaesthetic was effective, and Jon didn't feel a thing. Each
tooth that was extracted came out swiftly and easily, with
practically no gum left to hold it in place.

'Well done, Jon,' I said after a few minutes. 'All finished.'

'Sorry to have been so much trouble,' Jon said.

He smiled with gratitude and relief. His periodontally poorly
teeth had given him pain for the last time.

With Jon's permission, I called his mother once more, to report
on his well being and give her my personal thanks.

AGORAPHOBIA

What happens if we feel even more uncomfortable about going
out than we do about visiting our dentist? How do we get help

then? Of course, our GP's may be able to refer us for CBT to help with our agoraphobia, but meanwhile, the pragmatic answer to our dental dilemmas may lie in only visiting the dentist when our need is greatest. This may not fit with the ideal of preventive dental maintenance but if crisis management is more realistic, then perhaps it is kinder to work within our current capacities than to shame ourselves for our limitations.

A BRIDGE TO NORMAL LIVING

'You've got to perform a miracle,' Veda said.

'Miracles are tricky,' I said.

'You can do it. You did it last time,' Veda said.

'That was when you only had two front teeth missing. Now you want me to replace four upper teeth with a plastic bridge,' I countered.

'Yes,' Veda said. 'You have to do it. I don't trust anyone else.'

'I've done it with porcelain and precious metal. Canines are strong, they support the span. But I've never tried resin filling material on a gap that long. I just don't know if it's strong enough,' I said.

'You can do it,' Veda repeated.

'How about a denture?' I asked.

'No. My denture didn't feel normal, even after two years. And remember what it did to my gums? That's why we did the first bridge, to get rid of my false teeth. And I hate having something that comes out of my mouth and leaves me with a gap,' Veda said.

'A plastic bridge *is* cheaper than a permanent bridge. A permanent bridge can't be justified with the condition of your gums,' I said.

'Yes. I know my teeth are all going to fall out eventually. It would be too much money for something which might not last long,' Veda said. She repeated my own arguments back at me, pleadingly.

Veda was a former champion Eastern European weight lifter, now working in a biscuit factory. Her mother had lost all her teeth by the age of 40 years. Veda smoked heavily and had no intention of giving up the habit. Her teeth were loose from the ravages of her genetic inheritance and progressive smoking related gum disease. Her lateral incisors had drifted down and outwards. They now sat in pools of infected soft tissue, her weakened jawbone having long ago disappeared.

Veda suffered from agoraphobia, and only visited when her teeth were in a dire condition. She refused referral to a gum specialist, preferring palliative care.

'You might not get much wear out of the plastic bridge either. Your gums will continue to worsen, and you will lose more teeth,' I said.

'I'd like you to do what you can for as long as it works,' Veda said.

'I wouldn't be able to give you any kind of guarantee,' I said.

'I understand,' Veda said.

I offered Veda a written treatment plan for a six-unit immediate resin plastic bridge to replace her upper front teeth. I specified there was no guarantee for the work. Veda signed without hesitation. I sighed, and countersigned the plan.

Veda made herself comfortable. I numbed and removed her loose lateral incisors with the old attached bridgework; a few seconds work in their terminal state. The sockets, only millimeters deep, quickly clotted. We checked Veda's teeth for colour matching. We acid cleaned her canines, applied clear plastic bonding liquid, and placed a veneer of hardwearing resin over each canine surface.

With my nurse passing me resin and a light curing unit at alternate intervals, I fashioned new teeth to replace Veda's missing ones, attaching them to the canine veneers. I placed, shaped, sculpted, set and polished the resin to recreate Veda's smile. I continually checked the profile, contour and length of the bridge, blending it with the architecture of Veda's existing teeth and gums. I adjusted the surfaces of the bridge to ensure harmony with all the ways Veda could bite her teeth together. I confirmed there were no sharp or rough edges. Finally, I checked and flossed Veda's new bridge.

Over two hours had passed since Veda first sat in the dental chair.

'I'm not going to give you the mirror yet, Veda,' I said. 'I want you to go and have a cigarette.'

I do not usually exhort my clients to smoke. My nurse looked at me quizzically.

'Thank you,' Veda said.

While Veda smoked in the back garden, I explained to my nurse that the last time I did bridgework for Veda, she burst into angry tears at the end of treatment, declaring the work to be nothing like her familiar, comfortable denture, and leaving Gentle Dental inconsolable.

A week later, she returned, contrite and grateful, explaining the relationship between nicotine withdrawal and her outburst.

This time, we were managing the nicotine levels in her bloodstream proactively.

'I'm ready,' Veda said when she returned.

I passed Veda the mirror.

She smiled. And smiled again, more broadly.

'It's wonderful! I look better than before!' she said, hugging me tightly.

'Thank you,' I said.

Veda declined the offer of an appointment for regular preventive care. She said she would contact us when she felt the need. Last time it was years between visits.

As time passed, Veda returned intermittently for as much dental hygiene as possible while she had further loose teeth removed and bonded bridges added to replace them. Eventually, she gave up smoking, first by switching to herbal cigarettes, then by cutting down, and finally by cutting them out completely. Even without regular visits, Veda's determination and our occasional preventive messages had improved the quality of her now tobacco free life.

If our agoraphobia is so severe that we simply cannot leave home, or if, like Mrs Lonsdale, we are housebound for other reasons, a domiciliary dentist may be the answer to our prayers. This may take some research to arrange but may be the only way to gain emergency dental care for ourselves or an incapacitated loved one.

DOMICILIARY DENTISTRY

I didn't usually do home visits, but this was an exception. Mrs Lonsdale had had a wonderful new denture made, in time for her only daughter's wedding. There was just one small catch. Mrs Lonsdale needed her remaining four decayed and diseased teeth out before the denture could be fitted.

Mrs Lonsdale was in a wheelchair, slightly dementing, morbidly obese and largely housebound. Her daughter, Jennifer, explained that it would take three fit men to get her mother out of the house on the wedding day. If I finished her dental care at home it would be an enormous blessing.

Against my own usually agoraphobic judgment, in a moment of compassion, I agreed.

Jennifer greeted me at the door of the family home.

'Mum's in the lounge. She knows you're coming,' she said.

I walked through to the front room.

'Who are you?' Mrs Lonsdale asked.

'I'm Kathy, your dentist,' I said.

'I'll leave you two to get on,' Jennifer said. 'I've got to pop out. I'll be back in an hour.'

She kissed her mother on the cheek and left. I felt very alone.

Mrs Lonsdale and I eyed each other. I smiled.

I'll just make your teeth nice and numb first, and then we'll take them out and put your lovely new denture in,' I said.

Easy. Just like that.

'No,' Mrs Lonsdale said.

'I've come especially. It won't take long,' I said.

'No,' Mrs Lonsdale said.

I paused. Reassessed. I didn't know how long I could stay, trying to persuade Mrs Lonsdale to have her teeth out, whatever her daughter's wishes.

'How about if I just put some of the magic jelly on to numb the gum. You don't have to have the teeth out, but just see how the jelly feels first, then decide.'

Mrs Lonsdale nodded, and opened her mouth. I applied the topical anaesthetic before she could change her mind.

I waited a minute or so.

'It's time to put some magic liquid in to numb the teeth,' I said.

'No,' Mrs Lonsdale said.

'How about if I just do one spot, and then you decide about the others?' I asked.

Mrs Lonsdale nodded, and opened her mouth again.

'Doing great,' I said, withdrawing the anaesthetic cartridge.

Mrs Lonsdale looked at me silently, her mouth closed again.

'Ready for more?' I asked.

'No,' Mrs Lonsdale said.

'Just one more?' I asked.

Mrs Lonsdale nodded, and opened her mouth.

Gently, patiently, with a series of 'justs', 'one mores', and, 'you're doing greats', I completely numbed all Mrs Lonsdale's premolars. With her specific consent and assistance, I delivered her teeth safely and painlessly, and fitted her new dentures.

I heard the front door opening. Jennifer came into the lounge.

'How are you doing?' she asked me.

'All done,' I said. 'Your mum's done really well.'

I gave Jennifer instructions for aftercare. Jennifer looked at her mother.

Mrs Lonsdale smiled.

'Mum, you've got teeth!' Jennifer said.

'Yes,' Mrs Lonsdale said.

Two months later, I received a thank you card with a wedding photo enclosed. Mrs Lonsdale sat in her wheelchair, smiling with her new teeth, resplendent in her best dress and hat, centre front of the bridal party.

DISEASE AND DEATH PHOBIAS

Those of us with phobias about ill health or death avoid dentists because of our fear of receiving unwelcome news or our fear that somehow, every visit might be our last. Whilst this is entirely logical (most of us don't want to be ill or killed) the reality is that regular visits and early detection of mouth disease helps keep us and our teeth alive and happier for longer. If this hasn't convinced you, dentists are also now required by law to keep up to date, equipped and trained to manage medical emergencies and resuscitation in general practice.

MR ROOSEVELT 'DIES'

Mr Roosevelt, a very stiff and upright man, was seated in his usual formal fashion in the lounge. He never spoke to the staff, nor volunteered any information about himself, even after many years of visiting the practice.

On this occasion, I asked him if he would like a glass of water – it was very hot outside. Mr Roosevelt, (I never dared address him by his first name, Edward) gave no response. I asked again, a little more loudly, in case he hadn't heard over the quiet hum of the air conditioner. No response.

People often have to grab my attention, or at least my arm, before I hear them when they speak to me, particularly if I am focused on something else. Mr Roosevelt was elderly, and maybe becoming hard of hearing. Still, I hesitated to lay a hand on his arm out of politeness and respect, but he seemed strangely unmoving and I was becoming concerned.

Finally, I moved to be directly in front of him and spoke clearly.

'Mr Roosevelt, would you like a glass of water?' I asked.

There was no reply. Mr Roosevelt's eyes were glazed and he had a fixed stare on his face. He was unmoving and unresponsive. I did not hesitate to touch Mr Roosevelt now. I shook him by the shoulder, firmly.

'Mr Roosevelt, are you okay?' I asked.

I felt for a pulse. There was none. I could not see his chest moving. I put my ear close to his mouth. I could not feel or hear him breathing.

'We have a Code 9!' I called to my nurse.

This was the signal to call an ambulance and begin CPR – cardiopulmonary resuscitation, to try to maintain oxygen levels and blood circulation around Mr Roosevelt's body until the ambulance workers arrived.

Without ceremony, and thanking God there were no other clients in the lounge at the time, I dragged Mr Roosevelt onto the carpeted floor, made my best attempt to loosen his tie, checked his mouth was clear and tilted his head back. I began giving two breaths over his open mouth alternating with thirty chest compressions, one per second.

My nurse dialed 999 and summoned an ambulance. She ran and fetched the Automatic External Defibrillator (AED), the emergency drug kit and the oxygen, stored close to hand in the clinic. Mr Roosevelt stirred, coughed and tried to sit up.

'You've had a collapse Mr Roosevelt, but you're going to be fine,' I said, cradling teddy, Mr Edward Roosevelt, in my arms.

We went through yet another simulation, always practicing our roles to keep our resuscitation routine down to under three minutes, the critical interval for restoring oxygen flow to the brain of a collapsed person.

Teddy, our mannequin, has lived to assist us in many more training exercises. Fortunately, in three decades of dental practice I have never had to resuscitate a client. But at three monthly intervals and whenever we have a new member of staff, our team practices so that just in case we ever do need it, there is every chance of a good outcome for our living clients who would like to stay that way.

DRUGS PHOBIA

Perhaps you are worried about the effect of chemicals and drugs on your body. Ideally, we all seek to minimize the amount of unnecessary foreign substances we put into our bodies to safeguard our health. All conscientious dentists routinely take a thorough medical and general history from us before commencing treatment and avoid anything we might be allergic or sensitive to. In Evelyn's case this led to a challenging solution to her dental problem and a surprising revelation.

SAY NO TO DRUGS

'I can't have anaesthetic,' the young woman said.

'But you need an extraction. It's got huge decay. That's why you have toothache,' I said.

'I'm really sensitive to all chemicals,' the woman, Evelyn, said.

'I could give you antibiotics to control the spread of infection, but that won't fix the decay. You'll be back with pain in the future,' I said.

'I can't have antibiotics. They upset my system,' Evelyn said.

'I could root fill and fill the tooth, but it's a non functional wisdom tooth, it wouldn't make sense to keep it, and you'd still need local anaesthetic,' I said.

'No chemicals, they mess with me badly,' Evelyn said.

Evelyn looked at me, pale and tearful. She had not eaten or slept in the twenty-four hours prior to her appointment. Her grossly decayed wisdom tooth had kept her in constant pain.

'Please get rid of the pain,' Evelyn said.

'It needs to come out. The tooth needs to come out,' I said.

'Can you do it without anaesthetic?' Evelyn asked.

I looked across at my dental nurse. Extractions without anaesthetic were not part of my repertoire. I doubted they were company policy at the northwest London practice where I worked as an associate. I doubted that there was a company policy on the matter. There wasn't much call for extractions without anaesthetic as a rule. Ever.

My dental nurse raised her eyebrows.

'How about if I use a plain anaesthetic without adrenaline?' I asked.

'No chemicals, I have a really bad reaction to chemicals,' Evelyn said.

'If I refer you for treatment with sedation or general anaesthetic, you'll still be in pain until the tooth is out,' I said.

'I can't take another day of pain, and sedatives and general anaesthetics are drugs,' Evelyn said.

I looked at Evelyn.

'Please, take it out,' she said.

'No anaesthetic?' I asked.

'No anaesthetic,' Evelyn said.

'I'll be very quick,' I said.

My nurse raised her eyebrows further, and passed me a pair of upper wisdom tooth forceps.

'My nurse will support your head, and I will count to three,' I said.

Evelyn nodded.

'Ready?' I asked.

Evelyn opened her mouth.

I placed the forceps deep on the neck of the rotten tooth. 'If you can't be painless, be quick,' I reminded myself, in the words of one of my very pragmatic dental school oral surgery tutors.

'I'm going to count to three,' I said aloud.

Evelyn waited.

'One, two...' I said.

I pushed, twisted and pulled on the tooth, delivering it in one movement.

'It's out,' I said.

'Thank God for that,' Evelyn said.

'How are you?' I asked.

'It feels better already,' Evelyn said.

'That's because the pressure from the infection is gone,' I said.

'Thank you,' Evelyn said.

'Look after yourself today, please rest,' I said.

My nurse handed Evelyn an information sheet with aftercare instructions.

Evelyn scanned the leaflet as we cleaned up around her.

'No smoking?' she said, surprised.

'No smoking. It can cause serious problems with healing. You didn't mention you were a smoker when I asked you earlier,' I said.

'I only smoke socially or when I'm bored or stressed,' Evelyn said.

'How many would that be a day at the moment?' I asked.

'Only about 15 a day…when **can** I have a cigarette?' Evelyn asked.

'Not for at least a day, preferably longer,' I said. 'I'm obliged to mention that 15 a day is considered moderate to heavy smoking. Would you like a booklet on giving up?'

'Sure,' Evelyn said. She seemed resigned.

My nurse's raised eyebrows had disappeared under her fringe. She passed me Evelyn's notes.

I wrote 'smoker' on the front of Evelyn's record card, right next to where I had written the words, 'no chemicals, drugs or anaesthetics', in bold capitals.

EMETOPHOBIA

Most of us would agree that vomiting is unpleasant to watch, let alone experience, and would consider a phobia about vomiting (emesis) quite reasonable. If you detest, abhor and fear vomiting what happens if this terror gets in the way of receiving dental care?

HAIR RAISING

Judy's mother asked to speak to me privately before her daughter's appointment.
'Judy hates coming here. She hates being in all doctor's and dentist's surgeries in case someone vomits,' Mrs Wright said.

'Why do you think that is?' I asked.

'When she was five, she broke her arm, and while she was waiting to be seen in the hospital, someone vomited in front of her. She's been like it ever since,' Mrs Wright said.

'Can't say I blame her,' I said.

'She's ten. She should be over it by now,' Mrs Wright said.

'Ah. Phobias have a logic all of their own. They're designed to protect us from harm. I imagine Judy associates vomiting with pain and fear and injury since her trauma,' I said.

'Well, she needs her teeth checked. She's still got baby teeth and her adult teeth are coming through,' Mrs Wright said.

'I'll see what we can do,' I said.

Judy was sitting quietly, too quietly, with her father in the lounge room. I called her in to join her mother and I in the clinic.

'Hi, Judy,' I said.

Judy looked up at me from beneath her long fringe, suspiciously.

'Your mum says this is not your favourite place in the world, so I want you to let me know any time you need a rest, or to cough or swallow while I'm looking at your teeth. Just put your hand up and we'll stop straight away. And if you need to spit out, just use the little bowl on your left hand side.'

Judy pushed her fringe back slightly.

'I've cleared my super dentist diary just for you today, so no one else will be in the lounge room while you're here,' I said. 'This time is just for you.'

Judy looked at me directly.

'What are you going to do?' she asked.

'We're just going to look at your teeth and count them,' I said.

I patted the dental chair. Judy looked undecided.

'Hop in,' I said.

Judy climbed into the chair. She was small for her age.

'Here's Pandy. He's going to help us count your teeth,' I said.

Judy smiled for the first time as she held Pandy, our panda bear. I counted and charted all Pandy's teeth and then Judy's.

'Beautiful! I said. 'You have both your adult and your baby teeth at the moment. It's called the mixed dentition stage and it's absolutely, perfectly normal,' I added for her mother's sake.

I gave Judy a certificate, sticker and prize for being so helpful. She went back to the lounge room where her father was waiting.

'Look, Dad, look what I got!' she said.

'How did you do that?' Mrs Wright asked.

'I reassured Judy that she wouldn't see anyone else during her visit, that she had control over the procedure and that it would be totally painless. It's what we do for all our clients,' I said.

'Well, it certainly worked like magic today,' Mrs Wright said.

'Although Judy is ten, when she's confronted with her fear, it's possible that she is emotionally five again, the age when she was first frightened by the sight of vomiting. When Judy goes to the doctor's or a hospital, you might consider taking a book or game to distract her while you wait. You can be supportive of her fear and her progress in overcoming it at the same time. It might be more fun for her and she can still hide behind her hair when it all gets too much,' I suggested.

Mrs Wright shook her head.

'Well, I never,' she said, as she left the room.

VERTIGO

Those of us who have wrestled with vertigo know what it's like to have the wobbles, literally and metaphorically, when we go to the dentist. What may help us here is a combination of empathy and practical attention, as was the case for Cassie.

THE WOBBLES

Cassie, a middle aged sales manager, was so phobic about the dentist she would only communicate in emails with the practice at first. My practice manager, a qualified counsellor and psychotherapist, is gifted at making people feel good about themselves. He made contact with Cassie by telephone and arranged a strictly non-clinical, no obligation discussion designed to learn more about her and encourage her trust and confidence. After this gentle introduction, I was invited to join the meeting.

Speaking in front of and on behalf of Cassie, my practice manager then described her as interesting and special, rather than scared, scary, silly or stupid, all of which she'd heard from previous dentists. Her last visit to a dentist was six years ago. She'd had a filling which was unexpectedly painful, and when she was repositioned upright in the chair, had experienced a sudden severe attack of vertigo.

Cassie vividly described how the young and recently qualified careworkers in attendance had stood back, leaving her to crawl out of the surgery on her hands and knees, only calling her back into their clinic to pay her account. The dizziness was completely debilitating, leading Cassie to suffer bedridden days and long-term job loss despite her formerly good employment record.

Having experienced the horrors of vertigo myself, I could identify with both her suffering and her phobia, always a good place to start. We worked out that we would avoid any sudden movements which triggered Cassie's attacks by always allowing the dental chair to move independently of her, slowly helping her into position at her own pace and never allowing her head to drop below her feet.

All good. With Cassie's agreement we moved onto a full check up, cleaning, oral hygiene instruction and fluoride treatment, all without incident and with lots of love.

But oh, Cassie's teeth. A combination of time, sugar and cigarettes had been too much for her upper teeth, which were literally decayed to gum level in some areas and falling out in others. I felt sad telling Cassie that she would be losing all the teeth in her upper jaw, and relieved when she said that that was what she had expected, and even wanted, now that their appearance was so bad that she always covered her mouth with her hands when she smiled.

So, a week later, I removed/extracted ('delivered' in Gentle Dental speak) all Cassie's upper teeth, with loads of anaesthetic and hand holding. I was quick. Cassie was, thankfully, understanding and forgiving. 'It had to be done', was her comment.

It was amazing to see the improvement in Cassie's appearance, health and spirits as her work progressed. Working with our highly skilled denturist, Cassie had a new immediate denture fitted as soon as the last of her upper teeth were removed. Even with the effect of the local anaesthetic, she looked wonderful.

I passed Cassie a mirror to reveal her new smile.

'You look like Audrey Hepburn with your new teeth,' I exclaimed.

'Oh my God, so I do,' she agreed, beaming.

ARACHNOPHOBIA

How do we manage our dental visits when we are the owners of more than one phobia? What if, for example, we hate dentists and spiders, and not necessarily in that order? Sometimes, it helps to hand over our fears to others more willing or able to manage, as Anna's experience illustrates.

HARD TO IMPRESS

'Can you guarantee to fix my tooth in one appointment?' the woman on the telephone asked.

'I never guarantee anything without seeing the tooth first, but I do help most people get out of trouble in one appointment,' I said.

'I don't ever want to have to come back again,' the woman said.

'Okay,' I said.

'Which type of x-rays do you use?' the woman asked.

'We get the big ones that go right around your head and show all your teeth and jaws, the orthopantomographs,' I said.

'What about bitewings?' the woman asked.

'We like to have the big OPT's first because we get much more information with less radiation exposure that way. But if we need small x-rays for detail, we can always get them too,' I said.

'How will you tell if the tooth would be better off with a filling or an extraction?' the woman asked.

I spent another five minutes discussing the criteria for restorative versus extraction treatment planning. Every answer seemed to lead to another question.

'You know a lot about dentistry, and you ask intelligent questions,' I commented.

'I am a dentist myself,' the woman said.

'Wow. That's great. Where do you work?' I asked.

'I don't work as a dentist. I'm a medical secretary, I work in the London teaching hospitals,' the woman replied.

'Oh,' I said.

'I gave up dentistry five years ago, soon after I graduated. I didn't like working on patients unless they were unconscious,' the woman said.

'Oh,' I said.

The woman, Anna, had heard about me from another of my clients, who recommended me. She booked an appointment for the following Monday.

'Welcome,' I said, when Anna arrived for her visit with her husband, Keith.

She shook my hand. My nurse offered various forms for her to complete. I checked her health history and other details.

'Would you like Keith to come with you into the treatment room?' I suggested.

'No. He can stay out here,' Anna said, indicating the lounge room.

'Okay,' I said, glancing at Keith. He seemed used to being referred to in the third person by Anna.

Anna settled into the dental chair, and we examined her mouth and teeth together as she looked in the hand mirror.

'It's the lower right wisdom tooth; it probably needs to come out. I realized after I spoke with you last week,' she said.

I checked my charting and her large OPT x-ray, obtained that morning.

'I think you're right,' I said. 'Would you like to have it done today, after we've cleaned your teeth?'

'Yes, please. I don't ever want to come back here again.'

I numbed Anna's lower jaw and gave her teeth a spring clean. I sat her up in the dental chair for a rinse.

I felt my nurse's hand gently on my shoulder. I looked up. My nurse pointed to a large brown spider in the corner of the treatment room.

I decided not to draw attention to the minibeast, and to deal with it after Anna had left the room.

Anna's attention had been caught by my nurse's hand signals, and she turned her head.

'Oh, my God, you have a huge spider in your surgery!' she exclaimed.

The moment for silent monitoring had passed. I got up, calmly apprehended the spider in my gloved hands, crushed it, and wrapped it in the gloves and a plastic bag. I disposed of it in the outside bin. I asked God for karmic forgiveness.

I scrubbed up, gloved back up, and took Anna's wisdom tooth out. It was painless, and took seconds.

Anna joined Keith in the lounge.

'It was amazing,' she said.

At last, I thought. She's ready to acknowledge my superior skill, extensive training, and comforting chair side manner.

'She chased and caught the biggest spider I've ever seen. She was so brave. I could never have done that,' she said.

Keith smiled. I smiled. Anna apologized for her earlier abruptness. I suggested a routine annual recall to keep her smile in top condition.

Anna got out her diary and we confirmed a time.

ALLERGY PHOBIA

In the case of people with allergies, it is particularly important to determine the nature of their hypersensitivity. A severe allergy reaction can lead to anaphylactic shock, a life threatening condition.

A near death collapse after an allergy to drugs used during medical treatment left Ella terrified. Subsequent care was aimed at identifying her allergic triggers and avoiding them entirely.

ALLERGIC TO DENTISTS

'Can you please tell me if the practice can deal with a very nervous patient with allergies who is sensitive to medication. I need extensive dental work but cannot seem to find a dentist that can cope properly with all of my problems.'

Ella's first email to Gentle Dental spoke eloquently of her concerns, fears and frustration.

A couple of emails and telephone calls later, Ella was sitting in the dental chair.

'I got really scared of dentists after I collapsed and had to go to hospital', she said.

'What happened?' I asked.

'My doctor tried me out on a new blood pressure tablet and I was very sensitive to it,' Ella said.

'And the fear of dentists?' I asked.

'I'm allergic to so many things, metals, drugs, foods, I can't even use certain toothpastes or shampoos... one of the dental anaesthetics you use isn't okay for me, and the last dentist I saw wouldn't treat me because of my blood pressure medication. I'm frightened I might collapse again, if you use something I'm sensitive to,' Ella said.

'Hmm,' I said.

Ella and I continued to build a more complete history of her health and social situation. A parent and carer for her young adult son and nephew, she worked full time in corporate recovery, travelled a lot, and could not by her own account, afford to be ill, let alone have any more near death experiences resulting from medical or dental interventions.

In addition to sensitivity and allergies to penicillin, shellfish, potatoes, nickel sulphate, contrast dyes used in imaging, oral contraceptives, certain metals, cosmetics, blood pressure medicines and toothpastes, Ella was also reactive to mepivicane hydrochloride, a local anaesthetic used in dentistry. Ella was a heavy smoker, whose high blood pressure was just controlled on low doses of a combination of the few drugs she could tolerate. Her sinus problems meant her nose was partly blocked, and she had a good gag reflex. Understandably, she preferred to be treated sitting more upright in the dental chair.

Ella contacted her previous and current health care workers, and we added a recent x-ray, dermatology report, and medical summary to her file.

'I'm happy to treat you with the anaesthetic that isn't like the one you react to,' I said.

'But the other dentist said he wouldn't. Why was that?' Ella asked.

'Some dentists think anaesthetic with adrenaline might raise blood pressure dangerously in people who already have high blood pressure, but actually, research has shown that's not the case. And the pain and stress of toothache or inadequate anaesthesia is probably more likely to put your blood pressure up,' I said.

'But what if I react? I'm sensitive to so many things,' Ella said.

'Good question. I won't be using optional medicines like topical numbing anaesthetic on the gum– we want to limit the number of chemicals you're exposed to. I will use the minimum anaesthetic dose for complete numbness, and I will use it slowly, so if you have any reaction, we will catch it early,' I said.

'I'm still frightened, after what happened with the doctor's drug that time,' Ella said.

'We also keep emergency drugs and oxygen on hand, we're trained in resuscitation, and the nearest hospital is literally three minutes down the road, which is why we keep hearing ambulance sirens outside,' I said.

'I know my teeth need attention,' Ella said.

'Not all those ambulance sirens are for us, by the way, but I wouldn't hesitate to call for assistance if I needed to,' I added.

'I've got to do it,' Ella said.

With just a little anaesthetic and maximum reassurance, we gently and uneventfully extracted Ella's troublesome decayed molar roots.

At her follow up visit, Ella reported her only difficulty was now slight sensitivity to a couple of metal containing oral hygiene products, which we easily substituted for rubber and plastic ones.

Ella's email arrived a week later.

'Just to let you know that I am fit and well. It is good to know that at long last I have finally found a dentist that can deal with my allergies and my sensitivities to medications etc. These issues resulted in my becoming almost phobic with regards to dentists. Most dentists do not take the time and trouble to investigate why their patients have become shy of a dentist's chair in the first instance. I shall see you in November without breaking out in a cold sweat. It will now become part of my routine rather than something to be avoided at all costs,' she wrote.

PAIN HYPERSENSITIVITY

'It's not that I'm phobic. I really do have incredibly sensitive teeth and gums. I feel every little thing, and it really hurts,' I hear you say.

Yes. And it's not fair. Some of us feel pain sensations at much lower levels of stimulation and at much higher levels of intensity. Some of us suffer with exquisitely sensitive teeth and dislike eating green apples, drinking hot or cold drinks, or breathing in cold air on a winter's day. Some of us have gums that feel extreme pain when our dentists insist on cleaning them. There may be many reasons why we feel pain severely which our doctors and dentists might help us with. In the meantime, our extreme sensitivity does not encourage us to relax as dentists blow cold air or water onto our teeth or probe our gums in the process of examining or caring for us.

The most important way to ease our journeys in this situation is to recognize and accommodate, with respect, our special dental needs. Then, as Nettie did, with the help of our chosen dentist and support team we can move forward.

A CRYING SHAME

'So good to see you,' I said to Nettie as I greeted her.

And it was. Nettie, a mother with two children, regularly made long trips across London to see me, a dentist 'she could trust'. Regularly, she cancelled her appointments because of severe menstrual pain. And regularly she rescheduled when the timing of her monthly cycle was more favourable.

'It's not good to see you. I'm dreading it,' Nettie said.

'We'll take it easy. You're in charge, we'll use our usual generous amounts and kinds of anaesthetic, and you can put your hand up and stop me any time you feel like a rest, for any reason,' I said.

'That's why I come here,' Nettie said.

Nettie climbed into the dental chair and tensely held her hands together. For the first time in the several years that we had known each other, Nettie was having a root treatment.

'This is a good decision. We are going to try to save that tooth for you,' I said.

'I do want to keep the tooth. It's right at the front,' Nettie said.

'We will do everything we can to save your tooth,' I said, applying numbing anaesthetic jelly to Nettie's gum. We waited and chatted as the magic jelly did its trick.

I slowly and carefully introduced anaesthetic liquid next to the tender premolar that had been giving Nettie so much trouble with toothache.

'You're doing brilliantly, Nettie,' I said.

Nettie held my nurse's hand and cradled our soft toy, Lambie, to her stomach with her free hand. I noticed her normally fair complexion redden. Tears slowly, silently rolled down her cheeks and into her ears as she lay on her back. My nurse patted Nettie's face and ears dry. Nettie did not raise her hand to stop.

'Are you okay, Nettie?' I asked as I finished the injection. I touched Nettie's upper arm softly.

'It didn't hurt at all. It just brings back so many memories,' Nettie said.

'Tell me,' I said.

'My mother was a dentist. She did all my dental care. When I needed fillings, she couldn't do them because it hurt so much, even with anaesthetic. She was angry with me. She said I wasn't a good patient and she sent me to a special doctor,' Nettie said.

'A paedodontist? A children's dentist?' I asked.

'Yes. I had to be knocked out for all my work. My mum said I was being difficult,' Nettie said.

'That must have felt very shaming, especially with your mother herself being a dentist,' I said.

'Exactly,' said Nettie. 'I wasn't trying to be difficult, it just hurt so much I couldn't do it.'

'Is it possible that you weren't difficult? Is it possible that you did and do feel pain much more easily and intensely than most people, and that's just the way you're made?' I asked.

Nettie looked at me, puzzled.

'After all, every month you suffer through really bad period pain. The doctors never found a reason for your pain, but it's there and it's real. Not every woman suffers like you do. You've learnt to manage your work and appointments around it, but it can't be easy,' I said.

'Yes,' Nettie said.

'I once treated a young man with excruciating toothache, one that kept him awake for hours on end. I thought it was a severe infection or nerve pain, but all he needed in the end was a simple filling and his pain disappeared. It happened to him twice, and each time his pain was identical. His dad was the same, he said. We thought it might have been genetic, his experience of dental pain,' I said.

'Really?' Nettie asked.

'Absolutely. And he's not my only client I can think of like that. Some of us just do have the dubious privilege of owning very sensitive mouths and bodies,' I said.

'Like me,' Nettie said.

'Yes,' I said. 'And you can feel sorry for people who don't feel pain easily or well. They can end up losing teeth because they don't get any early warning signals to get them to a dentist in time.'

'That's so true. I never thought of it that way. Thank you,' Nettie said.

Together, Nettie, my nurse and I carried on tending to Nettie's previously tender tooth until it was clean, sealed and filled.

I spoke to Nettie the following week and she was feeling much better. She thanked me again for healing her tooth - and for hearing her truth.

INTRUSION PHOBIA

A healthy disrespect for uninvited, foreign objects into our bodies is probably a good thing. Few would argue in favour of splinters, shrapnel, stabbings or unnecessary surgery for example. For those of us with an even stronger fear of intrusion, our phobia might put us off piercings, tattoos or cosmetic surgery. For some of us, however, our dislike of intrusion, appearing as a dislike of needles, probes, suction tubes, drills or even just lying back in the dental chair, might be due to a more serious underlying cause.

FOSTERING GOOD HEALTH

'I'm just going to lay the chair back like your bed at home,' I said as I reclined the dental chair for Georgia.

Georgia needed a couple of small fillings, and was there with her foster mother, June, a warm and capable woman in her late forties who had decided to take up fostering when her adult children left home. June stood to one side of the chair and held Georgia's hand.

'I'll just put some magic jelly on to numb your gum,' I said.

I put some local anaesthetic gel on a cotton roll and waited for Georgia to open her mouth.

'No!' Georgia said.

She let go of June's hand, sat upright in the chair and ran out of the room before any of us could move or reassure her.

'I'll go after her,' June said.

'Was it something I said?' I asked my dental nurse.

Five minutes later, June was back, alone.

'Georgia is waiting in the lounge,' June said.

'Is she okay?' I asked.

'She is, but she got a fright when you lay the chair back and wanted to put the cotton roll and gel in her mouth. She said it reminded her of her father's sexual abuse of her when she was eleven,' June said.

'Oh,' I said. I flinched inwardly at my ignorance and poor choice of words. Suggesting that the dental chair was 'like her bed at home', usually reassuringly familiar to children, might have been an additional trigger to her flashback.

'I'm so sorry,' I said.

'Don't be,' June said. 'She's been with me three years now, since it was reported, and she hasn't been able to talk about it. This has helped her.'

'That's brave of her to share with you,' I said.

'Yes, it is. Hopefully, it will help her work through her experience. She is very scared. Her father will be coming out of prison soon, and being heard, understood and protected will be critical to her sense of safety,' June said.

'Would it be possible to have a word with Georgia? I give you my absolute guarantee that I won't do anything at all without her full permission,' I asked.

'Sure,' June said.

When June returned with Georgia, Georgia was looking a little bit embarrassed.

'I'm sorry,' she said to me.

'I think it's me that needs to apologise to you,' I began. 'I'm sorry for not understanding your needs. So far, all I've done is remind you of difficult times and feelings you've had in the past. I'm really sorry. I would like to be able to help you better.'

Together, June, Georgia and myself discussed the options for Georgia's treatment, with the aim of minimizing any further trauma to her, physical or psychological. On the understanding that she could raise her hand and stop at any time, Georgia decided to have another try at having her fillings done by me with local anaesthetic.

Half an hour later, with brief rests for Georgia to catch her breath, swallow and spit out, we were finished.

'I'm so proud of you,' I said to Georgia, handing her a sticker, balloon and certificate.

'Thankyou,' Georgia said. She carefully peeled the backing off the sticker and placed it onto the lapel of her black leather jacket.

'Well done both of you!' June said.

Over the years, I saw several of June's foster children, but always remembered Georgia, and the courage she showed in healing from her experiences. June reported that Georgia chose not to maintain contact with her father after he left prison. She went on to study nursing and then midwifery, with the goal of delivering healthy babies into the arms of caring parents.

LOSS OF BODY INTEGRITY/ BODY IMAGE PHOBIA

As a survivor of many a bad haircut, I can empathise with others facing deleterious body changes. Unlike hair, however, damaged teeth do not grow back. The difference between a good haircut and a bad haircut might be three weeks, but a bad tooth intervention or injury can affect our looks permanently. If we have suffered dental disability to the point where we cover our mouths when we smile, feel constantly self-conscious during normal interactions or just don't feel 'whole' or 'ourselves', it is particularly important to find a dentist we trust to makeover our smile.

In some cases, the thought of having further treatment to fix our smiling sorrows might feel so challenging that we would rather settle for what we have than take what we feel might be any further unnecessary risks. That is our perogative.
There is no law that says we all have to have 'perfect' teeth or smiles whatever the pressures are to do so. Sometimes, simple acceptance is acceptable. Self-acceptance is a big forward step in being beautiful in the greatest sense of the word, regardless of what our society holds to be ideal at any given time. Sometimes, our 'defects' become our distinctive features if we carry them off with the confidence they deserve. When and if we decide to have cosmetic or restorative treatment for our smiles, we can work with a dentist we trust to achieve as satisfying an outcome as possible, knowing we are worthwhile, whole enough and good enough already, even before we make any changes.

'FEELING MYSELF AGAIN'

'How often do you vomit at the moment,' I asked Preeti, laying down my dental mirror on the examining tray.

'Not at all,' Preeti answered.

'Did you suffer any eating disorders or reflux in the past?' I asked.

'I never had any eating disorders,' Preeti said.

'Fruit, fruit juice, fizzy drinks, sports drinks?' I asked.

Preeti shook her head. 'I like water and milk,' she said.

'What about pregnancy and morning sickness?' I asked

'Pregnancy! I'm not even married,' Preeti said. She paused. 'Not that you have to be married to have children, but I wouldn't want to do that.'

'What about reflux?' I persisted. 'You know, where the contents of your tummy rise up into your mouth and you get a bit of sick or vomit in your mouth?'

'I don't think I ever had any of that,' Preeti said.

'That's interesting. The enamel on the back of your front teeth has dissolved away quite a bit. Sometimes people get that if they have acid in their mouths a lot, like with pregnancy morning sickness, reflux, or bulaemia, the vomiting eating disorder,' I said.

'Oh,' Preeti said. 'When I was a teenager, I was allergic to a lot of foods and I couldn't keep them down so there was practically nothing I could eat. I lost a huge amount of weight and my parents were really worried. I was vomiting a lot and my teeth wore away, that's why they put the white fillings on the front.'

'Oh,' I said. 'What happened?'

'The doctors couldn't find any cause for it and it went away on its own after about three months. I've never had it again,' Preeti said.

'Are your teeth sensitive these days?' I asked

'Not at all,' Preeti said.

I was pleased. If Preeti still suffered any undiagnosed allergy, eating disorder or gastric problem, then ongoing tooth sensitivity might be a sign that she was still ill and experiencing active tooth erosion.

'Okay. Well, I want you to use a high fluoride toothpaste as your regular toothpaste, and if any allergies, vomiting or tooth sensitivity come back, I want you to see your doctor again immediately,' I said.

'I hope not!' Preeti said.

We carried on checking and cleaning Preeti's teeth.

'All done,' I said, putting the dental chair back upright.

Preeti examined her teeth critically in the magnifying side of the hand mirror.

'I hate how my front teeth look. Is it possible to get rid of the stains at the edges of the white fillings?' she asked.

'It would be difficult. I've taken away as much as I can with the ultrasonic scaler and the polishing paste without actually drilling and redoing the white fillings,' I said.

'You know what I said about getting married?' Preeti said.

'Yes?' I asked.

'Bipen and I are getting married in four month's time. I never wanted anything done to my front teeth again before now because I am really worried it might make them look worse, but I wondered if you would be able to do anything?'

'What bothers you in particular?' I asked.

I felt a bit cautious, because even the slightest 'body dysmorphia', a disorder of self image, might mean that any change to Preeti's teeth would be greeted with disatisfaction. Preeti already looked dazzlingly beautiful by most people's standards. I hoped to establish the basis of her dislike of what seemed to me to be reasonable restorations.

'My own teeth were flatter and squarer. These ones look like round blobs stuck on my real teeth. They look okay, but they just don't feel like me,' Preeti said.

Preeti and I chatted about her options. Removing and replacing the existing white fillings (which could also stain at the edges and might look bulky), crowning the teeth (which would involve further tooth removal to make room for the caps) or removing the white fillings and creating and placing eggshell thin porcelain veneers which would offer the most permanent result with the least tooth removal.

'Although I would try my best, and my best is pretty good if I do say so myself, it would be irresponsible of me to promise I could make you look and feel exactly like you did before you had your problems and your white fillings,' I said.

'I understand. I'll need to think about it,' Preeti said.

'Sure. In the meantime, why don't you bring in some photos of yourself before you had the problems and the existing white fillings so I can see how your original teeth looked,' I suggested.

'Okay,' Preeti said.

When Preeti did bring in some photos of herself taken in her late teens, I could clearly see a difference in her appearance before and after her illness and fillings, exactly as she had described. We agreed, with additional disclaimers and cautionary management of her expectations on my part, to go ahead with cosmetic porcelain veneer treatment.

At her last appointment before her big day, Preeti said, 'I feel like myself again.' Some months later, I received a stunning photograph of Preeti in traditional Asian bridal wear, the beautiful, confident wall of her brilliant white smile complementing her shining red silk sari and her fabulous gold wedding jewelry.

POST TRAUMATIC STRESS DISORDER (PTSD)

A majority of general or dental phobias are, arguably, post-traumatic. A bad experience in the past may leave us with a legacy of fear or shame linked to specific aspects of life or dental care that we then seek to avoid.

One of my clients, for example, developed a severe dental phobia when she disembarked from an airplane and the steps weren't there. She fell to the tarmac, smashed her front teeth and needed a considerable amount of emergency treatment. For the better part of two decades she then avoided dentists and hospitals altogether unless she was in extreme need. The first part of our work together was bearing witness to her story and helping her to find the words to understand her experience, with empathy and acceptance. She went on to have her teeth crowned and cared for knowing that she and her story were in our minds.

When we experience a highly distressing event or series of events, our minds may have difficulty working through our thoughts and feelings, particularly if we feel shame, fear or isolation around what happened. Traumatic relationships, incidents, operations, complications, abuse, injuries, accidents or assaults, for example, can trigger PTSD, whether we were 'near death' at the time, or simply overwhelmed by a series of milder experiences of fear. PTSD is commonly associated with first hand experiences of trauma but also affects bystanders and those who respond to the event.

PTSD may be felt in our bodies as well as our minds, with body memories, out of body experiences and dissociation leaving us with a sense of disconnection between different parts of our minds, and our minds and our bodies. Symptoms of PTSD also include intrusive memories (re-experiencing the traumatic event in flashbacks), nightmares, increased anxiety and emotional arousal (hypervigilance), sleep difficulties, poor concentration, angry outbursts, and an avoidance of any reminders, or 'triggers' of the trauma – including visiting the dentist.

Untreated PTSD may lead to depression, anxiety, antisocial behaviour, and drug and alcohol misuse. This is not good for us, for those around us, or for our healing **SMILE!** journey. Our first requirement for PTSD recovery is finding a safe place to regroup. Sometimes this will be with the carefully selected dentist you choose to provide your dental care or a member of their skilled and loving team.

But what if the traumas that caused our PTSD were dental in origin? What if we haven't yet developed confidence in our chosen dentist? Going to any dentist, no matter how caring might retrigger our symptoms of PTSD and give us the opposite of an experience of safety and security. If we are too frightened at this stage to contact or meet dental folk in their practices or hospitals to talk through our experiences (let alone receive dental care), there are, thankfully, other ways forward.

Professional counselors and therapists who help with PTSD can be relied upon to ask us the right questions, listen with empathy, affirm our experience and our essential goodness and humanity and help us find the right words to understand what happened to us and how we felt about it then and now. No matter how long ago we were traumatised, simply being listened to can be enough to begin our healing process. Asking, 'What happened?' and 'How did I feel about it at the time and later?' is a good way to start our recovery, especially if we are able to share with others who have had similar experiences or who are empathic and supportive.

Professional counselors and therapists, like dentists and their teams, are ethically bound to treat our attendance, information and disclosures in the strictest confidence. They are able to help us and hear our stories because they are specifically trained for this very special work and because they have regular, ongoing supervision (again, completely confidential) with senior colleagues for their own professional guidance and support.

Successful talking treatment helps us remember and reclaim our experiences and feelings in a way that makes us feel better about ourselves. Finding a therapist can be as easy as calling or emailing a professional on a recognised directory or website (see RESOURCES for further details) or asking your doctor for a referral. Whether you choose a caring dental team member or a therapist to share with, you will know that you are not alone in your quest to heal from your history, and you can be proud of yourself for seeking the appropriate help to do so.

In Holly's case, below, although she had already shared the factual elements of her story in a court of law, it was the emotional understanding of every aspect of her experience that helped heal her dental phobia. There is nothing so terrible in this world that it can't be spoken of and worked through. Our experiences, feelings, thoughts and behaviours make us who we are, and we can be brave and honest in sharing and reclaiming these unique parts of ourselves and our life stories.

CHILDHOOD REVISITED

'I had a bad experience as a child with someone being stabbed in a dentist surgery and I struggle with any treatment. I have a broken tooth at the back of my mouth and would like an appointment', Holly emailed.

'I was so sorry to hear of your childhood experience at the dentist' I emailed Holly back. We reserved an appointment for Holly, confirming the details by email and 'phone.

Later that week, Holly arrived at Gentle Dental with her adult daughter, Seline. At Holly's request, Seline remained in the lounge room while Holly and I repaired to the treatment room for a chat.

'I wonder if you could tell me more about your childhood experience at the dentist,' I said.

'My mother married five times,' Holly began.

Holly's father was her mother's first husband, whom her mother divorced and summarily excluded from their lives.

'You won't be seeing him any more', she announced to Holly one day when she picked her up from school. Holly was six years old, and didn't see her father again until decades later.

Holly's mother remarried a dentist, divorced, and then married a man who sexually abused Holly.

When Holly was nine years old, her mother sent Holly to collect stepfather 3 from stepfather 2's dental surgery. Holly was greeted by the sight of stepfather 3 staggering out of the practice with blood streaming down his head and neck from scalpel blade injuries inflicted by stepfather 2, the dentist.

'I felt very scared', Holly said.

Stepfather 3 was cleaned up, and survived. He continued to abuse Holly, and went on to abuse at least one other girl, for whom Holly later gave evidence in court. In view of the time elapsed, lack of witnesses to his crimes, and his then eighty years of age, he was never imprisoned.

Stepfather 2, the dentist, was never convicted of assault. In all probability, he was enraged at stepfather 3 for Holly's abuse. It was assumed Holly's dentist stepfather avoided punishment because her sexually abusive stepfather would not have wanted the motive for the stabbing revealed.

'Your mother sent you to collect stepfather 3 from stepfather 2's surgery. She didn't go herself,' I pointed out.

'Yes,' Holly said.

'She must have known things might be heated between them, yet she sent you alone,' I said.

'Yes,' Holly said.

'You were her human shield,' I said.

'Yes,' Holly said.

I pointed out that Holly chose to protect her *adult* daughter from our detailed conversation despite Seline's awareness of the drama in broad terms. And as the deputy head teacher at a school for children with special needs, Holly was very active in nurturing and protecting vulnerable children.

'Yet your mother abandoned you many times. She removed your actual father from your life, she failed to protect you from your sexually abusive stepfather, and she placed you in front of the awful consequences,' I said.

'Yes,' Holly said.

'You were only nine years old,' I said.

'Yes,' Holly said.

'Is your mother still with us?' I asked.

'No. She married and divorced twice more after I left home. She died some years ago,' Holly said.

I took a risk.

'When my mother died, bless her, I felt relief,' I said.

Holly looked at me.

'She was delightful,' I said, 'but she was also incestuous, unboundaried, and fierce. I felt relieved when she was gone.'

Holly nodded.

We paused.

'Let's have a look at your tooth,' I said.

Out of the ashes of childhood traumas blighted with maternal fecklessness and neglect our alliance was forged.

Within a short time, Holly's irretrievably decayed and cracked wisdom tooth was painlessly delivered. It was smiles all round as I returned Holly to Seline and congratulated them on their courage and mutual support.

The following Monday I received a further email. The words 'lots of ill effects' leapt out from the screen.

I read on, only slightly reassured.

'Thank you for your kindness on Friday. I had no physical ill effects, but lots of emotional ones... am back at work and all good again today.'

At her next Smile Care Visit, Holly explained.

'It was so good to hear someone else say they felt relieved when their mother died. It's not the sort of thing you normally tell people,' Holly said.

'Yes,' I said.

'I spent the weekend reflecting on my marriage. My husband is lovely, but he doesn't do emotional support,' she said.

'Yes,' I said.

'My daughter broke off her relationship with a lovely man because she wanted to be with someone who would care for her emotionally and be strong for her,' Holly said.

I waited.

'I married my husband to get away from my family. I will stay with him, but he's not able to be strong for me,' Holly said.

'We all do have to grieve our losses,' I said, 'the ones from our childhoods, and all the ones our childhoods cause.'

'Yes,' said Holly.

Our next story involves a young man, a sales executive for a motor company, who went to great lengths to avoid any medical or dental experiences that triggered his post traumatic flashbacks.

NOT MY FAULT

Hadrian arrived for his dental visit in a late model prestige car that he parked on the forecourt of the dental practice. He unfolded his six-foot frame from the front seat, firmly closed the car's silver door and walked to our front door.

I opened the door almost as soon as Hadrian had rung the doorbell. I was already waiting in anticipation of his arrival. Overwhelmed by fear, Hadrian had not managed to make it this far on three previous occasions.

'I am definitely coming in and facing my fear, I do really, really appreciate you being so kind and I'm so sorry for constantly messing you about.

I have a huge fear of any doctor's surgery, dentists, hospitals etc ever since I was younger when my brother was involved in an accident and needed to go to hospital.

I so badly want to visit the dentist and for you to help me look after my teeth,' Hadrian had emailed after his last unsuccessful attempt to overcome his dental phobia.

Each time, I had sought to reassure him, inviting him to 'pop in' just to meet us if a full consultation was too challenging, and rescheduling his appointments for when he felt more able.

At last he had arrived. Without giving him too much more time to think, I gently guided him into the care room and invited him to make himself comfortable in the 'driver's seat', a subtle reminder that he was in charge. I asked him about his health, general and dental. I explained that I would count and check his teeth and gums and mouth, and that if he wanted to pause at any time, for any reason, he could raise his hand and that I would stop straight away. He nodded.

'Upper right eight, seven, six,' I began.

My nurse diligently charted Hadrian's teeth on his record.

'Five, four, three,' I continued.

Suddenly, I felt the dental chair shaking. I looked to see if there was anything wrong with the reclining mechanism or platform, but everything was in order and the shaking continued. Then I realized.

'I'm going to introduce you to a friend called Lambie,' I said to Hadrian, who was lying back with his mouth open, not breathing, and his whole body trembling with fear.

'If you hold Lambie on your lap, I will be able to see your tummy go up and down and I will know you are breathing,' I said.

'Thanks,' Hadrian mumbled.

My nurse passed Lambie, our cuddly, soothing soft toy, to Hadrian, and patted Hadrian's shoulder in between charting his teeth.

'You're doing brilliantly,' I said, putting down my mirror and probe. 'All finished.'

'I'm so sorry. I really appreciate you being so understanding, I'm really embarrassed of my fear because it's so irrational, I know everything will be fine but it's really nice to know that you understand,' Hadrian said.

'Why don't we have a little chat? Sometimes it helps to understand what causes our fears. You mentioned your brother had an accident when you where younger in your email. Can you tell me what happened?' I asked. We moved to the non-clinical side of the room.

'We were at a family picnic, I was about seven and my brother was nine years old. He fell over running down a hill and broke his leg,' Hadrian said.

'What happened then?' I asked.

Our parents were over the other side of the hill and couldn't see us. My brother wasn't moving. I shouted for help, but it was ages 'til they came. They took him to hospital and he had his leg in plaster for weeks,' Hadrian said.

While he was speaking, Hadrian seemed to be looking down or over my shoulder, anywhere but into my eyes.

'What did you think when you saw him lying there?' I asked.

'I thought I caused it. I dared him to a running race, but the hill was muddy and he didn't have the right shoes on. When he lay there not moving, I thought he was dead and that it was my fault. Mum and Dad didn't say anything, but I thought they blamed me,' Hadrian said, looking at me.

'I can see how you might have thought that at the time,' I said. 'And I can also see how you wouldn't want to go near anything medical now in case it reminded you of that fear and shame.'

'Yes,' Hadrian nodded.

'Okay. Just for my sake, just imagine that you now have a nine-year-old son of your own whose has broken his leg falling down a hill trying to win a running race with his little brother. What are you going to say to his little brother?' I asked.

'I would ask him if he was okay and give him a big hug?' Hadrian said.

'Yes. Anything else? What if he said it was his fault, that he dared his brother to a race, or even that he knew the hill was slippery?' I asked.

'I would say he was doing what brothers do, they compete with each other, and that his big brother would have been able to look and see what the hill was like himself before accepting the challenge. I would tell him I was proud of him for staying with his brother and calling us. I would say that I was sorry that I wasn't there for him and his brother when they needed me,' Hadrian said.

'Yes, you would, wouldn't you,' I said.

Hadrian nodded slowly.

'How do you feel now?' I asked.

'Better,' he said.

'That's good,' I said.

We scheduled a time for Hadrian's next visit. Over the course of a couple of weeks, Hadrian had a decayed wisdom tooth removed, a super spring clean of his teeth for the first time in ten years and a custom made smile whitening kit which lifted his teeth to a shade lighter than Hollywood white. He told his family about why he had hated the dentist in the past. He was not quite sure they completely understood, but he understood himself, and that was what mattered. He never missed another appointment for any reason.

In the next section of this chapter, we continue our quest to heal our phobias by examining some specific dental fears that may challenge our courage to move forwards with our **SMILE!** program. As always, we are free to take whatever feels true for ourselves and use it to empower us on our dental adventures.

DENTAL FEARS

DENTAL PAIN PHOBIA

It seems sensible to be wary of pain. After all, pain hurts. However, most of us are willing to tolerate a little pain (or even a lot) if we feel it is for a good cause – think of childbirth. Sometimes pain is a fairly annoying side effect of getting to where we want to go, but one we grudgingly put up with. Any one who has started exercise after a long break or had tattoos or piercings can identify. But this does not necessarily mean we like pain. Or, indeed, and perhaps especially, dental pain.

Dental pain is different – and not in a good way. For a start, dental pain is in our heads, a highly sensitive and literally 'thoughtful' area of our bodies right near to our brains, the seat of our consciousness. This is an area that is not easy to 'escape' from mentally or physically when pain is felt.

Then, there is the lack of control we experience over whether, when, how much and for how long we feel dental pain when we offer ourselves up for dental care. Not all surprises are good surprises, and unexpected dental pain is one of them. Think about how much easier it is to remove a splinter from your own body, when you are in control, compared to when you allow someone else to do it for you. If we can't control when, how long and how intensely we experience a discomfort for, it definitely amplifies our helplessness, anxiety and yes, pain.

So, what can we do to manage an understandable fear of dental pain? One of my clients, Rita, developed a dental phobia after a traumatic dental experience involving severe, prolonged, unanticipated pain. As was the case for Rita, it is essential to create a calm atmosphere where you have control, with hand signals in order to be able to stop and communicate with your dentist at any time. This helps us overcome our fears and reclaim our ability to look after ourselves at the dentist.

SECRET COURAGE

Rita had a badly broken down tooth that was giving her pain. She knew she needed it out. She had come to her first appointment prepared for an extraction, with Matthew, her boyfriend, for support. We agreed the tooth was too decayed to save and that an extraction would be wise, the sooner the better, before the pain and infection worsened.

Rita was relieved and grateful to find a dentist (me) willing to offer an emergency appointment to fix the problem. There was just one even bigger problem.

'I hate needles', Rita said.

Rita was absolutely phobic about dental injections. At the age of 8 years, she had had an unexpectedly painful dental injection that had gone on for an excruciatingly long time. The dentist had continued despite her obvious shock and pain, and her mother had told her to, 'Get on with it'.

As an adult, Rita had all her previous dentistry carried out with general anaesthetic, where she could be 'put to sleep'. We discussed all the options for treatment this time, weighing up the risks and benefits of each, including referral for similar support with sedation or general anaesthetic.

But Rita wanted her tooth out today. She had seen my website, and she wanted to improve her ability to receive dental care while conscious, an experience she trusted me to provide.

'Sure', I said.

Rita, Matthew, my nurse and myself, all trooped into the care room (I never say 'surgery'). Rita sat herself in the dental chair.

She was literally shaking with fear. I deployed 'Lambie', one of the soft toys I use for just such occasions. With Rita holding Lambie tightly, my nurse patting Rita's arm, and Matthew stroking her hair, I applied 'magic jelly', a topical anaesthetic gel to numb the gum before injection.

Building trust is a delicate and crucial process. Fear of prolonged or unexpected pain was a significant factor in Rita's phobia. I asked Rita to indicate to me with a raised hand if she wanted me to stop, and promised to do so immediately, even if she just wanted to, 'rest, cough, swallow, or comment on the weather'.

I used the 'tell, show, do' technique to avoid surprises, informing and demonstrating to Rita at every stage what I was about to do. Some people prefer not to know or see what is being done for them, and that is respected. Other people like the reassurance of explanation and advance notice, and Rita clearly benefited from this.

Rita was encouraged to breathe, focus on wriggling her toes, and to feel a deepening relaxation spreading from her toes, up her legs, and throughout her body as she relaxed and breathed ever more deeply during her care.

Rita stopped shaking, and relaxed her rigid hold on Lambie. With the support of my team, I gently and slowly numbed Rita's jaw with a local anaesthetic injection in her mouth. I spoke soothingly and hypnotically to Rita. The offending tooth was carefully delivered in two sections while Matthew and my nurse held their posts supportively.

Once finished, I congratulated Rita and assured her that she would not miss the tooth at all, which we then examined carefully. Rita noticed how much bigger and more rotten it was than she had imagined. Rita also took the opportunity to look at and touch the anaesthetic needle, which she declared was much smaller and finer than she had thought. She was delighted to have coped so well with treatment, and said she now felt confident to have future treatment with local anaesthetic only, a great step forward in practical and emotional terms.

'I'm such a coward. I should have come much sooner', Rita chastised herself.

I reminded Rita that her fear and avoidance was the result of the childhood trauma over which she had been powerless, not because of any weakness on her part, and that a phobia is a logical way to protect oneself until a sense of safety is assured.

Then I reminded Rita that she was not, in fact, afraid of needles, well, at least not all needles. She looked at me, puzzled.

'A picture paints a thousand words', I said, pointing to the beautifully wrought tattoos on her arms, silent tributes to her courage and determination.

NEEDLE PHOBIA

Not many of us willingly line up for an injection, even when we know it will do us good, like vaccinations, or do others good, like donating blood. There are increasingly alternatives to needles for pain free dental care, such as wands (micro pressure anaesthetic devices) or hypnalgesia (using hypnosis for dental anaesthesia). But sometimes, old fashioned trusted dental injections reach the parts that others don't and provide us with the security of effective localized numbness and comfort while our dentists happily tinker away at our teeth. Our needle phobias, a very specific type of intrusion phobia, can affect any of us, and hamper our efforts to finesse our smiles, whatever our age or station in life.

COURAGE UNDER FIRE

'Whatever you do, don't show me the needle,' Peter said.

I assured him we wouldn't. We would apply some magic jelly first to numb the gum before putting his teeth to sleep. And we would hold his hand.

An ex-military man, Peter worked as a security consultant for national government and foreign countries facing terrorist threats and domestic disturbances. At age forty-two, six foot four inches in height, and weighing fourteen stone in lean body mass, Peter seemed an unlikely candidate for a dental needle phobia. Dental needles are thin, beveled, flexible, and designed to cause minimum tissue disturbance. They are tiny in comparison to big, strong men.

But size doesn't matter in many areas of life, and most especially when it comes to needle phobias. Needle phobias are a great leveler. Young or old, male or female, truck driver or artist, the mere thought of an injection can turn a normally confident person into an avoidant coward.

And dental injections are the worst. They are intraoral, inside a physiologically and psychologically loaded part of the body. Our mouths are the seat of our first relationships; we depend upon them for feeding and survival. They have huge social and sexual value. We eat, drink, talk, smile and make love with our wonderful mouths. Our sensitive and delicate mouths are centre front of our heads and necks. Right near our brains. There is no getting away from the sensations and thoughts we experience here.

For all the above reasons, it makes absolute sense for us to look after our amazing mouths, the source of life and love for each and every one of us in so many ways. And thus the eternal dilemma for those of us who want the best of dental care with the least of intrusion, least of all from needles.

I never say the 'N' word at the chairside. The closest I come to referring to needles is when I ask my nurse for 'LA', or local anaesthetic. We always keep needles, holders and carpules of anaesthetic covered or hidden, discreetly out of view. My nurse passes me LA behind the back of the dental chair, and I move the anaesthetic to the side of the client, before placing it carefully in their mouth.

I introduce anaesthetic slowly and gently in the area already numbed with topical anaesthetic gel– the magic jelly. I tell clients if they, 'might feel it just a little bit', in the interests of mental preparation and managing expectations.

As I work, and as the anasthetic works, I make helpful suggestions and affirmations, a form of hypnosis, if you will.

'You're doing really well.'

'Your teeth are going nice and numb.'

'You have excellent anaesthesia.'

Most people, even those of us with needle phobias, manage very well indeed.

'You've done brilliantly,' I said to Peter at the end of his treatment.

'As long as I don't see anything, I'm fine,' Peter said.

'Take care,' I said, as Peter walked to the door.

'I'm off to advise the armed forces on controlling and de-escalating riots now,' he said.

I thought of Peter's safety and of some of the photos he'd brought in over the years of himself and colleagues in full combat gear, battle ready.

'Whatever you do, don't show me the pictures,' I said.

BLOOD PHOBIA

Of all our fine and fancy fears and phobias, some people consider blood phobias to have the strongest genetic basis. Blood phobias, it is suggested, are designed to help us survive injuries by ensuring that we faint at the sight of blood in order to ensure our limbs are level and our blood loss is slowed, keeping us alive for longer, or at least until first aid arrives. Others would say that blood phobias are literally a bloody nuisance, especially when they get in the way of our ability to care for others and ourselves.

WORK EXPERIENCE

For many years, I have had the privilege of hosting work experience students at my practice, ranging from untrained teenagers to graduate dentists working towards UK accreditation. Tiny, sixteen year old Seema was one of the former. As was my custom, I had invited her parents to meet me and see where she was working. Mr and Mrs Parti arrived just as Seema was watching me complete a particularly thorough spring clean for a new patient who had not been to a dentist for over twenty years.

'I'll bet this is more than you expected to see,' my client, the 76 year old Mr Webster said, looking at Seema.

Seema looked pale and worried.

'You've done brilliantly, Mr Webster. Help yourself to a rinse,' I said.

I returned the dental chair to its upright position. My nurse filled the rinse cup with fresh water. Mr Webster picked up the cup, filled his mouth with water and swished firmly. Then he spat out, into the chairside spittoon. The white, glossy enameled porcelain turned red with the blood of over two decades of untreated periodontal disease.

Seema swayed where she stood as her legs buckled.

'Catch her!' I shouted to my nurse.

'I'm so sorry about this,' I said to Mr Webster.

'Happens to women in my company all the time,' Mr Webster said.

My nurse lay Seema flat and administered first aid as she gradually returned to consciousness.

'Excuse me,' I said to Mr Webster, as I went to call Seema's parents.

'Mr and Mrs Parti, lovely to meet you,' I said.

We all shook hands.

'Just to let you know that Seema's had a small fainting episode, but she is recovering well,' I said.

'Where is she?' Mr Parti asked.

'She's in the clinic now,' I said.

Mrs Parti ran to the clinic door and up to Seema, who was now sitting up and looking much better.

'Seema, are you okay?' Mrs Parti asked.

'Blood, Mum,' Seema pointed at the spittoon by way of explanation.

'I'm so sorry about this. Work experience student,' I said to Mr Webster quietly.

'We were all young once,' Mr Webster said.

Mrs Parti looked over at the dental chair as we were speaking. Her face turned pale and her legs buckled. I reached her just in time.

'Oh, dear,' I said.

I asked Mr Webster to excuse me once again. I helped Mrs Parti out to the lounge room and sat her on the settee next to her husband where she began to recover. Seema followed quietly on the arm of my nurse.

'It's the blood, they don't like the sight of blood,' Mr Parti explained.

My nurse took over the care for our very patient patient, Mr Webster, and arranged his next visit.

'I promise you it's not always like this,' I overheard her saying.

With Seema's soft spoken input, Mr Parti, his wife and I discussed alternative careers to healthcare for their much loved, blood phobic daughter.

TOOTH LOSS PHOBIA

We need to lose teeth like we need a hole in the head... and for some of us a lost tooth **is** a hole in the head, one that stops us from feeling whole and good enough. Like the experience of losing any other part of our bodies, losing a tooth or teeth can be a painful reminder of other losses, our fallibility, our advancing years and our mortality. If we have had extensive dental work done in the past, it can feel even worse if it fails, leaving us worrying that nothing in our lives is reliable or good enough, including ourselves. Despite advances in modern dentistry that make replacement teeth a realistic option for most of us, a tooth loss phobia can still leave us feeling 'less than' when it strikes. Sometimes, ironically, our fear of tooth loss is so great it stops us taking effective steps to look after our teeth properly, actually making it more likely that we will lose our teeth, a self-fulfilling prophecy if it happens.

TOOTH LOSS PHOBIA

Mariam finally found the courage to visit after emailing us via our website and asking if she, 'could have a chat with the dentist before her appointment and have her hand held'.

'Yes and yes!' was my reply.

When she arrived, Mariam explained she was too frightened to brush her teeth for fear they would drop out, particularly around the porcelain veneers she had on her upper front teeth, the most visible part of her smile.

She explained that she was literally terrified of the dentist, and worried about criticism, having been 'told off' by so many dentists in the past. She regretted the condition of her teeth and 'knew they were awful'.

After a compassionate discussion of her situation, Mariam agreed to let us look at her teeth and work out a way forward, together.

With Mariam in the dental chair, aka the 'driver's seat' in gentle dental speak, we conducted an examination, using mouth mirrors only. Her teeth were covered in old, years old, deposits of plaque and calculus, untouched since the veneers were first placed. A couple of premolars had decayed to the gumline.

X rays revealed an impacted (stuck) wisdom tooth in an area of infection.

But Mariam's biggest challenge was tooth loss phobia, which prevented her from cleaning her teeth, and with cruel irony made their decline and loss ever more likely.

Some people decry the use of 'labels', which they fear stigmatise and further shame people with the conditions they describe. My experience is that knowledge helps overcome fear, shame and isolation. And that with the naming or diagnosing of a condition, a conscious awareness of it, the first step in its management or treatment, begins.

In fact, it was a relief for Mariam to have a way to describe her experience. She was not bad, lazy, ignorant or irresponsible. She was suffering the consequences of an undiagnosed and untreated tooth loss phobia. We agreed to a gentle cleaning of her teeth and a referral to our local hospital oral surgeons for extraction of the awkward wisdom tooth and the decayed premolars.

With some trepidation, and the power of veto at any time using a raised hand to communicate, Mariam allowed me to scale, polish and floss all her teeth, including those with veneers.

Nothing fell out. Mariam watched in a hand held mirror as we worked, and as the accretions of years of fear and neglect fell away. At last Mariam looked and felt the youthful 38 years old that she was.

When Mariam relapsed into self criticism and self shaming, I reminded her that she was not a coward, and that I was very proud of her courage. I pointed out that many of our clients with dental phobias have children, and they all say that childbirth is easier than dentistry.

> Mariam laughed. She had four sons, all under the age of ten. The next day I received a lovely email, with an attached photo of her beautiful boys, all smiling.

DRILL/ULTRASONIC PHOBIA

Why would anyone like having their teeth drilled or ultrasonicated? All that noise, vibration, and dare I say it, pain. We may also have fears about dentists slipping and cutting our mouths – after all, they are using instruments that can cut hard tooth enamel in our mouths. In reality, this is an extremely rare event; dentists use 'finger rests' to prevent slippage occurring when we move, and tiny mouth mirrors, suction tubes and tissue guards to protect our lips, cheeks and tongues while they get on with looking after our lovely smiles. But there are many good and varied reasons to have fears or phobias around dental instruments and they all need to be heard, understood and respected if our conscious dental care is to be successful.

> ## BESPOKE DENTAL CARE
>
> 'I've brought my own CD to listen to while you work,' Kandy said.
>
> She presented me with a compilation disc of soothing yogic background music.
>
> 'How are you feeling today?' I asked.
>
> 'I still hate it here, but I want to keep my teeth,' Kandy said.
>
> Kandy was a woman in her fifties with an eclectic career portfolio reflecting her diverse skills and talents as a psychotherapist, masseuse and chef.
>
> Over several appointments and using a method of trial and error, mainly my errors and Kandy's trials, we worked hard to find

thoughtful ways to treat Kandy's teeth and gums. If I ever needed to do fillings for Kandy, wherever possible I used enamel and dentine bonded white fillings, where no anaesthetic injections or drilling would be required. Now, I used fine hand instruments to lovingly clean every surface of Kandy's teeth – Kandy hated ultrasonic scalers of any kind, with their high frequency whine, copious water jet and obligatory suction accompaniment.

With hand signals and 'commercial breaks' for Kandy to cough, swallow or simply rest and check in, we completed a thorough cleaning of her teeth. The gum disease that she had struggled with in the past was well under control.

'Your gums and teeth are really stable now,' I said.

'Thanks to you,' Kandy said.

'All of us,' I said. 'Team effort.'

'I was a mess when I first came here,' Kandy said.

'You were very frightened,' I said.

Kandy nodded.

'The first thing I liked about you was that you said I could raise my hand and you would stop at any time,' she said.

'Yes,' I said.

'And you did,' Kandy said. 'And you never caused me any pain.'

'It is a magic trick. For some reason people prefer not to have pain. It's the first thing we have to get right,' I said.

'But you talked with me. You listened to me. When I told you how my mother treated me as an object for her own pleasure when I was a child, you heard me. You understood that that was why I didn't like to be touched by anyone, especially not with instruments,' Kandy said.

Kandy had bravely shared the reasons for her fear of all things dental at her very first visit.

'That's true. It's perfectly possible to have dental care without understanding, but it makes life so much easier when you do,' I agreed.

'I feel better about myself and my fears knowing you do understand,' Kandy said.

As she spoke, Kandy reached into her tote bag on the settee. She pulled out a small, square package.

'These are for you,' she said. 'I know you don't eat sugar, so I made them with fruit puree instead.'

Kandy handed me a presentation box of beautiful, bespoke chocolate cookies, individually and lovingly prepared, with me in mind.

HALITOPHOBIA

Some of us are convinced we have bad breath even when we don't, and no amount of reassurance from family and friends will convince us otherwise. When we suffer from this condition, also known as halitophobia, we can end up avoiding social contact and talking, smiling or even exhaling near others for fear of causing offence or suffering shame. If our halitophobia is part of other conditions causing delusions, we may need a once over and specialist referral from our GP's to get us all the help we need. Our dentists, however, are ideally placed to give us a thorough professional assessment to ease our anxieties and get us back into the self confidence and social loop.

FRESH BREATH CONFIDENCE

Jasu, a woman in her thirties, seemed to have great difficulty opening her mouth. Cleaning her teeth was a challenge, and even the examination was tiring as I struggled to carefully inspect her mouth with a mirror. I imagined how much more challenging and exhausting it must be for her. But she didn't have any obvious jaw joint problems or areca chewing habits.

For the uninitiated, areca, also known as betel, pan, sopari, tulsi, guthka, masala, etc. is a plant product widely chewed by people in our Asian communities. It comes in commercial packets or rolled up in leaves and mixed with tobacco and occasionally spices or sweeteners. It is delightfully sedative and euphoric. But it is also addictive and causes mouth scarring (oral submucous fibrosis, or, OSF) and mouth cancer.

One of the early signs of OSF is loss of the ability to 'open wide'. But my client didn't chew areca. Nor did she suffer from arthritis or trauma or any other problems in her jaw joints. She could easily and painlessly open her mouth 4cm (or 4 finger widths – try it on yourself and see) when asked.

My client and I talked. I explained that I noticed she had some difficulty opening her mouth, but there didn't seem to be any obvious clinical cause. Did she have any ideas?

And here the first clue emerged. Jasu said she felt selfconscious because she had bad breath. This was news to me. As I shared with her, I'm usually highly aware of halitosis. I have a good sense of smell, even with a facemask on, and can smell periodontitis (gum disease) from a distance.

So I whipped out my Fresh Breath Questionnaire (FBQ) and waited while Jasu patiently read every question and ticked the answers she felt were true for her. The FBQ is a natty little diagnostic, educational and management tool. I put it together after surveying research on halitosis and working out that causes of bad breath all fall into simple categories, for example, oral, medication related, and psychosocial causes, among others.

Then it was easy. Jasu did not have any diseases or habits relating to bad breath, and no one had ever told her she had bad breath, not even her husband or previous dentists. In fact, she was quite conscientious about cleaning her teeth. I reminded her that I would be the first to tell her if I thought she had bad breath. In view of the complete lack of any other evidence or explanation for her fear of bad breath, I shared my diagnosis of halitophobia with Jasu.

Jasu said that when she was growing up in India, she didn't have floss, and felt unable to clean her teeth properly. She felt shame around this, and imagined that she had bad breath, a fear she still carried today.

I reassured her that this was absolutely no longer the case, but that closing, covering and reducing her mouth opening, smiling, speaking, kissing and lovemaking would definitely be affecting her enjoyment of her life now.

We talked about how easy it is to imagine other people's body language as shying away from bad breath, when in fact they might just be polite, reserved, or just trying to preserve a normal social distance from each other, especially in crowded situations like parties or public transport. And how important a full smile is, a valuable unit of social currency without which other people might not smile at us, leaving us living in a world of reflected gloom. And how halitophobia helped her deal with fear, shame and shyness in the past. And the impact of halitophobia on her social and intimate confidence today.

Jasu departed with an action list of new thoughts and behaviours to practise – identifying and accepting her halitophobia, a self chosen affirmation; 'I am the best', and last but not least, a reminder to SMILE!

Three months later Jasu arrived for her review appointment. Confident. And beaming.

She explained how her gums had improved with cleaning – she had found it difficult at first, but persevered, and was now using an electric brush and flossing daily. We fine tuned Jasu's home care with the introduction of little bottle brushes for interdental cleaning and gave her a loving and thorough scaling and polishing.

Most importantly, we talked. Jasu had carried out her own exercise in social anthropology since our first consultation, and observed how people naturally cover their mouths or lean back to protect their personal space in conversation – and not because they are repelled by the bad breath of the person who they are speaking to, as she had formerly imagined.

This, and her own improved oral hygiene, had effected a breakthrough in Jasu's life. She was now more confident in social situations, and able to smile at family and friends. She shared that friends had previously thought her aloof or even arrogant before getting to know her, because of her shyness and lack of smiling.

We talked about the next stage in halitophobia recovery; overcoming loneliness and improving her sense of connection with others. We discussed 'homework'; smiling at safe strangers and initiating conversation using compliments, sharing experiences, or asking questions. And practising saying 'no' graciously to unwanted attention or conversation rather than hiding behind the halitophobia generated shyness that had served this purpose in the past.

I admitted I was not sharing information as an authority, but as a fellow traveler on the road to social confidence. As a shy child who let my more outgoing twin sister do my talking for me, I am still getting over my sheltered beginnings today.

I disclosed that when I was dating, I had read a book called, 'The Shy Single', by Bonnie Jacobson, which was full of suggestions for people like myself navigating the world of social and intimate connection. I suggested another worthy tome, 'Watching the English', by Kate Fox, for decoding the rules of engagement on our little island.

Jasu and I agreed that CBT, our own organically developed version of it, seemed to be an effective means of overcoming both halitophobia and shyness. We discussed alternative treatments such as hypnosis, (helpful in phobias of traumatic origin), and psychotherapy, (to enable more fundamental personality transformation), but agreed that these might be less appropriate in this case.

And so, in the intimate confessional of the dental surgery, Jasu and I shared our strength and hope in shyness recovery. Jasu tells me she organizes large annual Diwali celebrations for her community, with displays of singing and dancing, and that she is one of the performers. And that she is delighted that her outgoing nature is now integrating with her feelings, awareness, thoughts and behaviours in one to one interactions. She said she felt she was 'becoming herself'.

We agreed to another Smile Care Visit in three month's time, at which appointment Jasu would bring photographs of herself on stage.

And here, just in case you were wondering, is the very same questionnaire (with my comments in brackets) that Jasu and I used to assess her fresh breath status:

FRESH BREATH QUESTIONNAIRE

To help us bring out the best in your smile, tick the statements below with which you agree:

Non-pathologic/physiologic causes of halitosis (bad breath):

1. I often eat onions, garlic, spices, cabbage, brussel sprouts, cauliflower, radish, durian.
2. I often eat meat, fish and/or milk.
3. I often drink alcohol.
4. I often drink coffee.
5. I often miss breakfast.
6. I often fast, miss meals, and/or diet.
7. I often do manual work and/or exercise.
8. I do a lot of speaking.
9. I breathe through my mouth.
10. I have a dry mouth (little saliva).
11. I notice I have bad breath and/or taste in my mouth when I wake up.
12. I notice I have bad breath in the late morning.
13. I notice I have bad breath mid-cycle and/or around the time of my menstrual period (women).

(Certain foods, drinks and proteins give culturally acceptable mouth odor in some circles but not others. If in doubt, avoid the food, or stick with your own tribe. Anything that causes dehydration can reduce the washout of odor causing bacteria, dead skin cells and gases from our mouths. Stick to safe limits of alcohol intake, eat regularly and drink water freely!)

Oral hygiene related aspects of halitosis:

14. I do not brush my teeth every day.
15. I do not floss my teeth every day.
16. I do not clean under my bridgework every day.
17. I do not brush/scrape my tongue every day.

18. I do not brush the roof of my mouth every day.
19. I notice a bad smell on my floss.
20. Sometimes my gums bleed.
21. I often get food stuck between my teeth.
22. My teeth are moving position and/or loose.
23. I do not leave my dentures out at night.
24. I do not clean my dentures every day.
25. My dentures are stained.
26. My last dental hygiene (professional cleaning) visit was over two months ago.

(Perform your recommended dental hygiene routine daily and well, with regular professional cleaning as prescribed by your dentist or hygienist.)

Oral/dental aspects of halitosis:

27. I often have ulcers, blisters and/or mouth infections.
28. I have had a tooth extracted in the last week.
29. I suffer from wisdom tooth infections.
30. I have gum abscesses.
31. My last dental examination was over 12 months ago.
32. I have decayed teeth.
33. My tongue is furry/coated.

(See your dentist at least annually, and for treatment of any mouth conditions that don't or won't improve on their own within three weeks– you know you want to!)

Drug related aspects of halitosis:

34. I am a smoker.
35. I chew areca (pan, tulsi, guthka, sopari etc.).
36. I take drugs/medications.

(Keep taking prescribed drugs and medications and giving up non-prescribed ones, with the support of your GP and pharmacist as required. Discuss any medication side effects, such as dry mouth, with your prescribers, and take little sips of water to keep your mouth moist and your breath fresh as needed.)

Ear, nose and throat aspects of halitosis:

37. I often have colds, sinusitis, catarrh (mucous), post nasal drip.
38. I often have tonsillitis.
39. I have tonsiloliths (calcifications in my tonsils).
40. I have asthma.
41. I suffer from hayfever.
42. I have broken my nose in the past.
43. I may have foreign bodies in my nose e.g. from childhood / past surgery.
44. I feel my bad breath is coming mainly from my nose passages.

(Any ear, nose or throat (ENT) condition that fails to improve of its own accord warrants a visit to your doctor and possibly a referral to an ENT specialist.)

General medical aspects of halitosis:

45. I am diabetic.
46. I suffer from stomach ulcers.
47. I have lung disease.
48. I have liver disease.
49. I have kidney disease.
50. My food often has or gives a fishy taste/I have trimethylaminuria.

(If you have any of the above conditions, your medical management is the first priority. If you have worrying symptoms of any kind see your doctor.)

Psychosocial aspects of halitosis:

51. I notice I have a bad taste and/or bad breath.
52. My partner/other adults have said I have bad breath.
53. The experience of bad breath is affecting my confidence.
54. I feel my life would improve if I had fresh breath.
55. I would be willing to change my behaviour in order to have fresh breath.
56. I have asked dentists in the past about my bad breath.

(This section of the FBQ is a handy indication of your awareness and motivation to manage any bad breath you may have. If you feel you have bad breath and no one else, including your dentist, agrees, you may have halitophobia.)

SUFFOCATION PHOBIA

Anything that gets in the way of our breathing is likely to cause us distress, to put it mildly. If we have suffered near death experiences as a result of smoke inhalation, choking, near drowning, sleep apnoea or asthma, for example, we may, in a completely understandable post traumatic way, prefer to avoid situations, like going to the dentist, where our airways are even partly obstructed. Hand signals will be invaluable here, letting our dentists know when we need a rest. Our breathing always takes first priority. Our natural, active gag reflexes are designed to protect us from suffocation. But they may also trigger our fear of suffocation.

A GOOD GAG REFLEX

'I'm so sorry, I've always been like this,' David said.

David, a forty three year old accountant, sat up in the dental chair, coughing and gasping. We had just completed his first dental examination in years. He had come in to have his teeth cleaned after his boss declared they would be taking and posting staff photos on the company website the following week.

'You have a great gag reflex,' I said.

'That's the first time I've heard it described like that. Usually it's a bloody nuisance. I've never been able to have my teeth cleaned without sedation,' David said.

'Well, that is always a possibility, but why don't we have a chat and discuss other options,' I said.

We sat in the non-clinical area of the treatment room and talked.

'Can you remember a time when the gag reflex started, or was it always like this?' I asked.

'I never liked going to the dentist, but when I was nine, I had impressions for an orthodontic plate. They put both trays with the gunge in them in my mouth while I was lying back in the chair. I couldn't swallow, I couldn't spit, my mouth filled with saliva and I couldn't breathe. I thought I was going to die. It went on for minutes,' David said.

'What happened then?' I asked.

'The dentist had a whole row of us kids in different rooms in different chairs. He and his nurse had gone on to the next one. I couldn't call out even if I tried,' David said.

'And then?' I asked.

'I was sweating and twisting, and trying to sit up when they came back. They told me to lie back down again. They took the trays out and sent me back out to the waiting room to my mum,' David said.

'What did your mum say about it?' I asked.

'She didn't say anything. I didn't tell her. There were all these other kids around with their mothers, and they seemed perfectly okay. I didn't want to make a fuss. They would have thought I was feeble,' David said.

'Well, I don't think you were feeble. These days, it's common knowledge that lying people back to take impressions can trigger a gag reflex. In the old days, treating people in assembly line fashion was considered smart practice for commercial reasons and to treat the large number of us needing NHS dental care. Leaving unsupervised children lying back with dental impressions in their mouths might well be considered negligent these days,' I said.

'Are you saying I'm not a wuss?' David asked.

'On the contrary. I'm saying you were very brave to survive the experience and still support the industry as an adult. I imagine that there may have been other kids who suffered the same as you and also didn't want to risk being shamed by saying anything,' I said.

David seemed thoughtful.

'If you took your nine year old child to the orthodontist to have impressions for a plate, what would you do?' I asked.

'I would want to be there in the room with him. I would ask the orthodontist to sit him up, give him a bowl to dribble into, and I would hold his hand. I would not leave him alone,' David said.

'Absolutely. And if he had a small mouth or a very active gag reflex, which they would notice after examining him, you would expect them to use smaller trays, one at a time, and to reassure him if he was in distress,' I said.

'You're right,' David said.

'So shall we try that for you when you have your teeth cleaned?' I asked.

'What do you mean?' David asked.

'Keeping you sitting up, letting you spit out or have a break whenever you want, and taking it in turns to let you pause and rest while we clean your teeth,' I said.

'You can do that?' David asked.

'I can do that. I make sure I allow enough time for my special clients to get the care they need, and all my clients are special,' I said.

'Okay, if you're sure I won't be keeping anyone waiting. I'll try,' David said.

For the next half hour, my nurse and I gently and thoroughly cleaned David's teeth. Using hand signals, speaking to him in our best bedtime story voices, keeping the chair more upright, and encouraging him to rest, spit or rinse whenever he felt like it, we managed to bring his smile back to its former, wonderful, shiny white glory.

'Have a look,' I said, passing David the hand mirror when we finished.

'Seriously!' David said. 'I will definitely have the cleanest, whitest teeth in the office when I get back to work!'

SWALLOWING PHOBIA

Is it possible to have a swallowing phobia? We have to eat and drink, don't we? How can a swallowing phobia be compatible with life? Yes, yes and with great difficulty, are the answers to these questions. Those of us with a mild swallowing phobia may find it almost impossible to take medication in tablet form, for instance. Those of us with a severe swallowing phobia may find it difficult to eat a healthy variety of nourishing foods or to accept dental care. Well meaning dentists, bless us, are constantly putting things in our mouths, which may be a challenge to those of us frightened of swallowing. But there are ways forward, gently.

STARVING

Lisa arrived at Gentle Dental with her grandparents supporting her, one on either side. Her eyes were glazed with fear. She had contacted the practice by email, writing, 'The [previous dentist] got very annoyed with me shaking, waving my arms and crying out...I am so petrified and feel that no one can help me. I am even scared writing this email. I feel as if my life is over and I am wary of trusting another dentist.'

In her early twenties, Lisa had had many hospitalisations for anorexia and panic attacks. She was terrified of eating. It would have been amazing if she weighed more than seven stone. Her grandparents, at their wits end, had been feeding her Mars bars to maintain her weight, such as it was.

Now Lisa's teeth had crumbled, overwhelmed by her diet of chocolate and fizzy drinks. A severe toothache meant she was even less able to eat, and her dental phobia meant she was unable to face treatment to fix her toothache.

A quick look at Lisa confirmed that she did indeed have a weight problem, and not of the overeating variety. She had not had breakfast that morning.

As a hard working professional, with years of training and multiple qualifications, I did what any other dentist would do in the same situation. I popped up to the kitchen and fetched Lisa a snack, a sugar free cereal and fruit bar. Call it my inner mother, I could not bear to see someone perishing of starvation on my watch.

As Lisa unwrapped the bar and began to chew at the edges, I talked with her grandparents about family life. Lisa was born prematurely, had her throat suctioned to clear her airways of secretions, and had practically choked as a tiny baby when efforts were made to feed her. She had never found eating easy.

While we talked, Lisa often paused to declare her throat felt blocked, like she was choking, and that she, 'couldn't swallow'. But she kept eating. Slowly. It took half an hour, with continual affirmations that she was doing a great job, and with reminders to keep breathing, but she did it.

Once the cereal bar had disappeared, we all settled in the care room (I never say 'surgery') and looked carefully at Lisa's mouth and teeth. With encouragement, Lisa allowed us to clean her teeth, a first in her experience of dental care.

I discussed what I felt might be the cause of Lisa's fear – her neonatal traumatic 'near death' experiences of airway obstruction, with a now unconscious association to the sensation of gagging and choking, which had generalised to feeding. All of which might best be described as a posttraumatic swallowing phobia, leading to anorexia, malnutrition and rampant caries (tooth decay practically everywhere).

Lisa and her family had travelled over 300 miles to the appointment. With the amount of work required, multiple extractions and fillings, further visits at Gentle Dental were impractical. We agreed to prescribe antibiotics as a holding measure and refer Lisa to her local hospital dental department, where her treatment could be carried out with general anaesthetic if this was indicated.

Not long afterwards, I received an email from Lisa thanking me for my support and confirming she had an appointment with the hospital the following week. When Lisa had visited us, she spoke with conscientiousness and concern about her work as a carer for elderly people. I hoped her experience might have restored some of her faith in the dental profession, and that she would be back to the work she clearly loved as soon as possible.

If, like Lisa, you are wrestling with the life threatening anorexic complications of your swallowing phobia, be brave and persistent. Keep asking for the help that you need to get better, and say 'yes' to the help that you are offered. As Riyad's story shows, we are never to young to start recovering from life's challenges.

SWALLOWING PHOBIA

Shorna despaired of her youngest child. At three years of age, he was smaller than all his friends and same age cousins, and did not eat well, despite being very active. Shorna had taken him to see various specialists who had eliminated ADHD (Attention Deficit Hyperactivity Disorder) or any other causes, and basically said the problem was behavioural. 'Put the food in front of him. He'll eat when he's hungry', they advised.

The last time Shorna had tried this, Riyad had not eaten for four days. She had tried star charts, praise, exhortations, cooking him special food, sending him to the laundry room at family meal times, and feeding him on her lap. At times he would chew endlessly, only to gag and spit out when his mouth became too full. Meal times had become a protracted battle ground, with her older daughter neglected, and Shorna and her husband feeling angry, alarmed and helpless.

Confusingly, Riyad would eat at nursery school and outside the home, and occasionally wolf down pizza if he was exceptionally hungry. Shorna, who seemed to be a conscientious and caring mother, had begun to blame herself, assuming Riyad must be acting out some terrible unresolved conflict by refusing to eat, and that she was a bad or at least seriously deficient mother.

Remembering Lisa, who had managed to eat a cereal bar at the practice despite her swallowing phobia, I wondered aloud with Shorna if Riyad might be having a similar experience, with the home environment triggering a pre-existing swallowing phobia. Shorna considered the similarities. Riyad had been born prematurely. It was likely that he had had his airways suctioned to keep them clear, a common practice in neonatal care. Her impression was that he was happy to have food in his mouth, but terrified of swallowing it.

When I examined Riyad, his mouth and teeth seemed perfectly healthy at least as far as I could literally see, to the level of his tonsils. He seemed happy and well adjusted, and very bright and active. Although Riyad was pre-cooperative in dental terms (four is considered the earliest age at which children begin to understand and follow treatment instructions) we did manage to have a little conversation with him about swallowing and eating.

With Shorna holding Riyad on her lap, and calling him back when he dashed off to play with his sister, we talked about the difference between how babies and adults swallow. I demonstrated how babies stick their tongues out to feed, and how grown ups keep their tongues in their mouths and how he might try that, and also swallowing twice with each mouthful, with water, to help food go down.

Shorna and I talked about how Riyad might need more time and even privacy to eat, so as not to increase his fear or shame about mealtimes at home. Shorna asked Riyad if he thought it would help him if he were able to eat on his own, and he nodded very firmly. I wryly suggested letting him eat at the dinner table while the rest of the family waited or dined in the laundry room, a gentle acknowledgement that Riyad's previous experience of mealtimes may have felt like punishment for something over which he had no conscious control.

But Shorna was already feeling guilt about her previous response to the situation and resolved to apologise to Riyad and try new techniques with love rather than exasperation. My heart went out to her. I shared about the times I had felt impatient with my daughter's behaviour before it was explained she had ADHD. And how I had seen many specialists before she was diagnosed and how things had improved for us after we received appropriate support, including parent coaching for me.

We talked about alternatives – referring Riyad to Great Ormond Street Children's Hospital, or trying hypnotherapy when he was older and able to respond.

Riyad and his sister left Gentle Dental with stickers and a prize. Riyad chose a soft teddy, a well earned present for being so good at the dentist.

SMILING PHOBIA

Do you cover your mouth with your lips or hands when you talk to people, or avoid showing your teeth when you smile? Do you offer a closed mouth smile in response to greetings or in photographs? Even on special occasions? Even in your graduation or wedding photos? Or maybe you avoid smiling altogether, in case any of your teeth are revealed. If we are so ashamed of our teeth that we stop smiling altogether, then we are putting our spiritual lives in serious danger. Smiling is a fundamental unit of social currency. Babies have an innate gift for smiling so their carers will look after them when they are helpless infants. (They also have annoying cries so we will do the same, but that's another story.) As adults, if we lose our capacity to smile for whatever reason, there is a danger that people in our lives will be less likely to smile back at us, leading us to live in a world of reflected gloom. Clearly, smiling is good for our mental and spiritual wellbeing, as our last story reveals.

SMILE POWER

Gina, a fashion buyer in her late twenties, had come in to see what could be done for her teeth. The first thing I noticed about her was her striking monochrome outfit. The second was not her teeth. In fact, Gina kept her teeth so carefully hidden by her lips or hands as she spoke, I could not tell if she had teeth. And she did not smile.

'Make yourself comfy in the driver's seat,' I said, introducing Gina to the dental chair.

Gently and tactfully, I checked Gina's teeth, gums, jaws and mouth tissues. She had a couple of badly decayed teeth and her front teeth were stained a very dark brown.

'You will need to have a couple of teeth out, the most badly decayed ones that I can't save,' I said.

Gina nodded sadly.

'I think I knew that,' she said.

'But I'm guessing your main concern is the staining on the front teeth. Do you drink a lot of red wine, tea or coffee, or smoke cigarettes?' I asked.

'It's the coffee,' Gina said. 'I love it. I have about ten cups a day to keep me going.'

'Oh. Okay. Apparently it's not good to have more than five cups of coffee a day. Would it be possible to alternate your coffees with water? That would keep you healthier and hydrated, and keep the staining down on your teeth at the same time,' I said.

'I'll certainly think about it. But is there anything you can do about the stains?' Gina asked.

'I can try and give your teeth a good spring clean, and then we can see what their natural shade is,' I said.

Gina and I agreed a treatment plan to fix all her teeth, hygiene and cosmetic problems. Over her next two visits, I removed her decayed tooth fragments and meticulously cleaned all her teeth. At each visit, Gina wore some combination of her striking black and white outfits.

'Have a look,' I said to Gina, passing her the mirror when all her treatment was complete.

'No thank you. I can't,' Gina said.

'Is that because you don't ever like looking at your teeth, or letting other people see them?' I asked.

'I'm too scared. They look terrible,' Gina said.

'Not any more,' I said.

Gina allowed her lips to pull back, ever so slightly, and then a bit more.

'Oh, my God, they're amazing, they match my white shirt!' she said.

Gina's teeth had gone from their deepest brown shade at her first visit to the lightest white on the professional shade guide, a youthful, bright A1. She inspected them carefully in the mirror.

'Oh, my goodness,' she said.

As Gina spoke, she still covered her teeth with her lips or hand.

'Gina, listen to me,' I said. 'Your teeth are beautiful, and you are beautiful. It's wonderful having a healthy, show stopping smile, but I want you to get full value from it. Will you make me a promise?' I asked.

Gina nodded.

'Don't agree until you've heard what I'm asking,' I said.

We both laughed.

'I suspect your shame about your teeth has given you a smiling phobia. I notice you hide your smile, even now, when it's looking amazing. It's become a habit that I suspect you have had for a long time and I want you to try and break it. I want you to practice speaking and smiling, first by yourself in the mirror, then in front of a photo of your loved ones, and then in front of your real friends and family – without covering your teeth with your lips or hands. It will take a conscious effort at first, but it is definitely worth it. You are worth it. You deserve to have smiles in your life,' I said.

'I will try,' said Gina.

The next time I heard from Gina was when I received a Christmas card from her.

'Dear Kathy,' she wrote, 'I just wanted to thank you so very much for making me feel so calm and relaxed. I have never experienced a visit to the dentist quite like it. You were so welcoming and friendly; my nerves just seemed to fade away. You cannot imagine how relieved I am to have finally found you. I am slowly but surely moving forward and starting to smile as well!'

So. I hope you are smiling now, too. You've come to the end of our collection of true tales of other brave and clever folk who overcame their dental fears and phobias to achieve outstanding oral health and sparkling smiles. If at first you don't succeed in getting the care you need, keep trying. This book is here to guide, support and inspire you on your way. And when you do take all you have learnt with you to your dental visits, be proud of who you are, your special needs and your own very special smile recovery story.

Chapter 10.

Enjoy!

We have completed our **SMILE!** plan to help us face our dental fears. Now is the time to look firstly backwards and then forwards, to enjoy the benefits of our brand new smiles.

Review

Congratulations! You've done it! After each visit to your dentist, and ideally with your dentist, take the time to debrief. Review your visit and think about what worked, how it compared to your expectations and what could be improved for use on your next visits. Yes, you heard me. Your next visits...

Repeat

Like cars and houses, our smiles need a lifetime of care and maintenance to look and work their best. Unlike cars and houses, our smiles are not as easy to replace when things go wrong. On the upside, our smiles are a part of ourselves, and something we use every day. Like ourselves, they are definitely worth looking after. So, keep up all the good work - **reserve your next appointment** (yes!) and continue with your excellent self-care. You deserve to enjoy a beautiful, healthy smile for life!

Reward

When you complete your journey to smiling loveliness, you deserve every certificate, sticker, prize, present, gold star, Well Done stamp and toothpaste sample your dentist has to give you. And more. Enjoy the inbuilt rewards of your triumphant smile transformation– eat, speak, smile and kiss (healthily, kindly and appropriately, please) to your heart's comfortable content.

Resist the temptation to conveniently forget the challenges you faced or to minimize your achievements; phrases such as, 'About time', 'I don't know what all the fuss was about', and 'Long overdue', do not belong here. Affirm yourself with a generous serving of praise. In your moments of relief and pride, smile at yourself in the mirror with your sparkling new teeth and say, 'You did it! So proud of you!' or words to that effect. A little self-congratulation goes a long way to reinforcing our new 'visiting the dentist' behaviours and looking after ourselves.

Finally, tell the world and share the love! Let one 'small' step for you inspire one giant leap forward for your fellow dentally phobic humankind. Recommend and refer other people in your life to your dentist. Offer to be part of their support team if you feel the call to do so. Tell friends, send emails or post cards, share testimonials and write blogs, tweets or posts about your brave and clever dental experience and smile upgrade. You did it! I am so proud of you!

RESOURCES

Organisations

Many organizations can help with information about dental fears and phobias and finding a suitable dentist (or therapist). How about trying:

General Dental Council
37 Wimpole Street
London W1G 8DQ
020 7167 6000
www.gdc-uk.org

British Dental Association
64 Wimpole Street
London W1G 8YS
020 7935 0875
https://www.bda.org

British Dental Health Foundation
0845 063 1188
http://www.dentalhealth.org

Faculty of General Dental Practice
35-43 Lincoln's Inn Fields
London WC2A 3PE
020 7869 6754
www.fgdp.org.uk

NHS choices
http://www.nhs.uk

Dental Fear Central
http://www.dentalfearcentral.org

Dental Phobia

http://www.dentalphobia.co.uk

British Association for Counselling and Psychotherapy
www.bacp.co.uk

Counselling Directory
http://www.counselling-directory.org.uk

Reading

Feeling academic? Try reading *Cognitive Behaviour Therapy for Dental Phobia and Anxiety*, Ost & Skaret, Wiley-Blackwell, 2013.

If you're looking for something a little more accessible, I found *Cognitive Behavioural Therapy for Dummies*, Willson & Branch, John Wiley & Sons, 2006, and *The Complete CBT Guide for Anxiety*, Shafran, Brosnan & Cooper, Constable & Robinson Ltd, 2013, much easier reads, although both were general rather than dentally specific in approach.

For those of us with a touch of PTSD, reading *Trauma: From Lockerbie to 7/7: How trauma affects our minds and how we fight back* by Professor Gordon Turnbull, Corgi, 2011, might be just what is needed to understand our experience and start our own journeys of dental recovery.

INDEX

Abscess
Affirmation
Alcohol
Allergies/hypersensitivity
Anaesthetic
- General anaesthetic (GA)
- Local anaesthetic (LA)
- Topical anaesthetic
Anaphylactic shock
Anchor

Anorexia
Antibiotics
Anxiety/fear/phobia
Apnoea/ Sleep apnoea
Appointments
Areca/ betel/ pan/ sopari/ tulsi/ guthka/ masala
Assault
Asthma
Attention Deficit Hyperactivity Disorder (ADHD)
Autistic Spectrum Disorders (ASD)
- Aspergers Syndrome
- Autism
Avoidance/delay
Awareness

Blisters
Body dysmorphia
Breastfeeding

Caffeine/ Coffee/ Cola/ Tea
Calculus/tartar
Cancer screening
Career
Care Quality Commission (CQC)
Celebrate
Chaperone
Childbirth
Cognitive Behavioural Therapy (CBT)
Communication
Confidence
Confidentiality
Coughing
Courage
Cosmetic dentistry
- Crown and bridgework
- Smile/tooth whitening
- Veneers
- White fillings

Cracked tooth

Deafness (hard of hearing)
Denial/doubt
Dentist
Dentures
Depression
Diabetes
Diet/nutrition
Domestic violence
Domiciliary dentist
Drowning
Drugs/prescriptions/medications

Ear, nose and throat (ENT) conditions
- Broken nose
- Catarrh/mucous
- Colds
- Foreign bodies in nose
- Hayfever
- Post nasal drip
- Sinusitis
- Tonsilitis
- Tonsiloliths
Eating disorders
- Anorexia
- Bulaemia
- Extraction
Ehlers Danhlos Syndrome (EDS)
Empathy
Exercise/activity

Faith/trust/spiritual approach
Fear/fear of diagnoses/fear of treatment/fear of additional
treatment
Finger rests
Fresh breath
Fresh Breath Questionnaire (FBQ)

Fun

Gagging/gag reflex
General Dental Council (GDC)

Halitosis (bad breath)
Hand holding
Health
Hygiene/ Hygienist/scaling and polishing/cleaning
Hypnosis/self hypnosis

Infection
Injection/needle
Inner child

Jaw fracture
Jaw joint problems/TMD

Kidney disease

Liver disease
Lung disease

Maintenance
Meditation
Menstruation/menstrual cycle
Mental health
Mistakes
Morning sickness
Mouth cancer/ oral cancer
Mouth infections
Mouth mirrors
Mouth opening

National Health Service (NHS)
Neck pain/problems
NHS Choices
Nicotine replacement

Night guard/mouth splint

Obsessive Compulsive Disorder (OCD)
Oral hygiene
- Electric toothbrush
- Floss threaders
- Fluoride toothpaste
- Interdental cleaning (floss/interdental brushes/sticks)
- Mouthrinse
- Plaque
- Tongue scraper
Oral piercings
Oral submucous fibrosis (OSF)
Oral surgery
Orthodontic wires/splint/retainer/archwires

Pain
Painkillers
Periodontal disease/periodontitis (gum disease)
Personal growth
Phobias
- Allergy phobia
- Agoraphobia
- Arachnophobia/fear of spiders
- Blood phobia
- Chemicals/drugs phobia
- Dental pain phobia
- Dental phobia
- Dental Phobia Questionnaire
- Disease/Death phobia
- Drill phobia
- Emetophobia/ fear of vomiting
- Halitophobia (fear of bad breath)
- Infection phobia
- Intrusion phobia
- Loss of body integrity/change of body image phobia
- Loss of control phobia/fear of powerlessness
- Mess phobia

- Needle phobia/injection phobia
- Pain hypersensitivity/phobia
- Smiling phobia
- Suffocation phobia
- Swallowing phobia
- Tooth loss phobia
- Ultrasonic phobia

Plaque disclosing tablets/solutions
Porcelain veneers
Post Traumatic Stress Disorder (PTSD)
- Antisocial behaviour
- Body memories
- Disconnection
- Dissociation
- Flashbacks/intrusive memories
- Hypervigilance
- Near death experiences
- Nightmares
- Out of body experiences
- Panic attacks
- Sleep/Sleeping/Sleep difficulties
- Trauma
- Triggers

Practice ritual
Precooperative
Pregnancy

Recommend/refer
Reflux/gastric disorders
Relationships
Relaxation
Removable orthodontic appliances
Resuscitation
Review
Reward
Root canal treatment/endodontics
Rubber dam

Saliva
Scaler
Schizophrenia
Sedation
- Inhaled (nitrous oxide/happy gas)
- Intravenous (midazolam)
- Oral (diazepam/temazepam)
Self acceptance
Self care
Self esteem
Self neglect
Sensitive gums
Sensitive teeth
Sexual abuse
Sexual health
Shame/fear of embarrassment
Smiling
Smoking/tobacco/nicotine/cigarette cessation
Smoke inhalation
Social media
Soft tissues/lips/cheeks/tongue
Soft toy
Special Care Dentistry
Sports guard/gumshield
Stomach ulcers
Stop signals
Suction tubes
Sugar
Suicide
Sun safety
Support team

Tattoos
Tender Loving Care (TLC)
Tissue guards
Tobacco
Tongue jewellery

Tooth decay/caries/holes
Tooth discolouration/staining
Tooth enamel
Tooth reimplantation
Tooth surface loss
- Abrasion
- Erosion
- Attrition
Trimethylaminuria
Tumour

Ulcers
Ultrasonic scaler

Vaccinations
Validation
Vertigo
Vertigo/dizziness/labyrinthitis

Waiting list
Water
Wellbeing checklist
Weight
White fillings
Wisdom tooth removal
Work experience

Printed in Great Britain
by Amazon